Defeating Diabetes with Evidence Based Strategies

Type 1, Type 2, and Beyond

Brenda F. Dozier

Table of content

Introduction

In the modern era, where the complexity of contemporary living appears to increase with each passing day, the prevalence of diabetes presents a daunting obstacle to the overall health and well-being of our society. Diabetes is a chronic disorder that is characterized by increased blood sugar levels. Diabetes is more than just a medical diagnosis; it affects every aspect of life, impacting individuals, families, and entire communities. Nevertheless, amid this widespread health concern, there is a glimmer of light in the form of evidence-based strategies that provide a road toward conquering diabetes, regardless of whether it is Type 1, Type 2, or any other variant.

The journey toward understanding diabetes and effectively managing disease takes more than simply clinical knowledge; it requires a holistic approach that covers the domains of biology, psychology, lifestyle, and society, all of which are intertwined with one another. Through the adoption of strategies that are supported by science, we give ourselves the ability to navigate the complex terrain of diabetes with precision and intent.

As we move on with our research, it is becoming increasingly clear that the story of diabetes goes well beyond the bounds of medical textbooks. It is closely linked to the decisions we make daily, ranging from the foods we eat to the activities we participate in, and it has a significant impact on the results of our health. As a result, the fight against diabetes transforms into a very personal undertaking that is guided by the ideals of self-determination, education, and perseverance.

In this introductory chapter, we lay the groundwork for a journey of discovery, a trip that will be fueled by the collective wisdom of medical research, the resiliency of individuals who are living with diabetes, and the unshakable commitment of healthcare professionals. Alongside one another, we go into the core of diabetes, dissecting its intricacies and locating the evidence-based strategies that offer the promise of a more positive and healthier future.

Join us as we go on this adventure to completely eradicate diabetes—not only as a medical disease but as a call to action for individuals and communities alike. Together, let us pave the path toward a world where diabetes no longer casts its shadow on the lives of millions, but instead, serves as a tribute to the victory of human ingenuity and resilience.

Understanding Diabetes Mellitus

Understanding Diabetes Mellitus is analogous to dissecting a multidimensional puzzle, where each piece holds essential information about this difficult ailment. At its core, Diabetes Mellitus, generally referred to simply as diabetes, encompasses a collection of metabolic disorders characterized by increased blood sugar levels over a sustained period. This seemingly harmless imbalance can exert substantial consequences on numerous human systems, making it necessary to appreciate its intricacies fully.

Diabetes Mellitus presents in numerous ways, with Type 1 and Type 2 being the most prevalent. Type 1 Diabetes occurs from the body's immune system wrongly attacking and destroying insulin-producing beta cells in the pancreas, resulting in a shortage in insulin production. On the other hand, Type 2 Diabetes is a combination of insulin resistance – where cells fail to respond appropriately to insulin – and relative insulin insufficiency.

The diagnosis of Diabetes Mellitus rests on the measurement of blood glucose levels, with fasting plasma glucose, oral glucose tolerance tests, and hemoglobin A1c (HbA1c) levels acting as main diagnostic techniques. Recognizing the signs of diabetes is similarly vital, covering frequent urination, excessive thirst, unexplained weight loss, exhaustion, and blurred vision, among others.

Beyond its clinical manifestations, Diabetes Mellitus carries substantial consequences for long-term health effects. Uncontrolled diabetes can lead to a multitude of consequences, including cardiovascular disease, neuropathy, nephropathy, retinopathy, and an increased risk of infections. Understanding these potential problems highlights the significance of proactive management and vigilant monitoring of blood sugar levels.

While the etiology of Diabetes Mellitus is multifaceted, certain risk factors predispose individuals to its development. These include genetic predisposition, lifestyle variables such as sedentary behavior and poor food choices, obesity, age, ethnicity, and certain medical disorders. Acknowledging these risk factors helps individuals to implement preventive actions and make informed lifestyle choices to decrease their chance of acquiring diabetes.

Grasping this Diabetes Mellitus involves navigating a landscape created by genetics, physiology, lifestyle, and environmental influences. By understanding the underlying mechanisms of this disorder and its potential repercussions, individuals can take proactive actions toward effective management and optimal health outcomes. In the chapters that follow, we go deeper into evidence-based techniques targeted at managing diabetes and encouraging individuals to enjoy healthier, more satisfying lives.

Differentiating Type 1 and Type 2 Diabetes

Distinguishing between Type 1 and Type 2 Diabetes is critical for understanding the subtleties of these distinct yet interconnected illnesses. While both varieties share the common trait of increased blood sugar levels, their underlying processes and management options differ greatly.

Type 1 Diabetes, often diagnosed in infancy or adolescence, originates from the immune system mistakenly attacking and destroying insulin-producing beta cells in the pancreas. This inflammatory response leads to an extreme shortage of insulin, the hormone responsible for controlling blood sugar levels. As a result, patients with Type 1 Diabetes require lifetime insulin therapy to control their illness adequately.

Conversely, Type 2 Diabetes normally develops in maturity, but it is increasingly diagnosed in children and adolescents due to increased obesity rates. This form of diabetes is characterized by insulin resistance when cells in the body fail to respond appropriately to insulin.

Initially, the pancreas adjusts by making more insulin, but over time, insulin production may decline, leading to a relative insulin shortage.

Distinguishing between Type 1 and Type 2 Diabetes includes examining numerous characteristics, including age of onset, autoimmune indicators, genetic predisposition, and insulin production levels. Individuals with Type 1 Diabetes frequently appear with rapid onset symptoms, such as extreme thirst, frequent urination, weight loss, and fatigue, whereas those with Type 2 Diabetes may suffer gradual onset symptoms and are often overweight or obese.

Diagnostic techniques, including measurement of fasting plasma glucose, oral glucose tolerance tests, and detection of particular autoantibodies, aid in discriminating between the two forms. Additionally, monitoring of C-peptide levels, a measure of insulin synthesis, can provide further insight into the underlying pathophysiology of diabetes.

Management techniques for Type 1 and Type 2 Diabetes also differ greatly. While insulin therapy is the cornerstone of treatment for Type 1 Diabetes, persons with Type 2 Diabetes may initially manage their illness via lifestyle improvements, including dietary changes, frequent exercise, and weight management. Oral drugs and, in certain situations, insulin therapy may be administered for Type 2 Diabetes if lifestyle measures alone are insufficient to control blood sugar levels.

Understanding the distinctions between Type 1 and Type 2 Diabetes is critical for efficient management and tailored care. By knowing the specific characteristics and underlying mechanisms of each type, healthcare providers can adjust treatment options to fit the individual needs of patients living with diabetes

Emerging Trends in Diabetes Management

Exploring the rising trends in diabetes management gives a window into the exciting breakthroughs and ideas driving the future of care for persons living with this chronic condition. As academics and healthcare professionals continue to push the boundaries of scientific knowledge, new technologies, and treatment methods are transforming the landscape of diabetes management.

One of the most promising advances in diabetes management is the development of improved glucose monitoring systems. Continuous glucose monitoring (CGM) devices, for instance, provide real-time data on blood sugar levels, allowing individuals to make timely adjustments to their food, exercise, and medication regimes. These devices offer higher ease and accuracy compared to traditional fingerstick glucose monitoring methods, enabling more proactive management of blood sugar levels.

Another rising trend is the incorporation of artificial intelligence (AI) and machine learning algorithms into diabetes management platforms. These sophisticated algorithms evaluate huge amounts of patient data, including blood glucose levels, insulin dosages, dietary habits, and physical activity levels, to create individualized suggestions for enhancing diabetes management. By embracing the power of AI, healthcare professionals may deliver targeted interventions that improve outcomes and enhance patient satisfaction.

Advancements in insulin delivery devices are also altering diabetes management. Smart insulin pens and pumps equipped with Bluetooth technology provide seamless contact with mobile devices, allowing for remote monitoring of insulin administration and dosing history. These gadgets not only ease insulin control for individuals with diabetes but also allow better communication between patients and healthcare providers.

Furthermore, regenerative medicine shows promise for the future of diabetes treatment. Stem cell therapy, for example, tries to restore beta cell function in persons with Type 1 Diabetes by replenishing insulin-producing cells in the pancreas. While still in the early phases of development, growing research in regenerative medicine gives hope for a potential solution for diabetes in the years to come.

In addition to these technological breakthroughs, a shift toward holistic and patient-centered treatment approaches is changing the future of diabetes management. Integrative treatments that address the diverse requirements of individuals with diabetes, including lifestyle variables, mental health, and social determinants of health, are gaining recognition as key components of complete care. By taking a holistic approach, healthcare providers can empower patients with diabetes to achieve improved health outcomes and improve their entire quality of life.

The developing developments in diabetes management signal a new era of innovation and growth in the field of healthcare. From sophisticated glucose monitoring devices and AI-powered decision support tools to regenerative medicine and holistic care models, these innovations give hope for a brighter future for persons living with diabetes. By staying current on these trends and embracing innovation, healthcare providers may continue to advance the standard of treatment for diabetes and pave the road for greater health outcomes for everybody.

Chapter 1

Type 1 Diabetes: Understanding and Management

Understanding Type 1 Diabetes is crucial to effectively managing this lifelong condition, which requires a distinct strategy compared to other forms of diabetes. Type 1 Diabetes, frequently diagnosed in childhood or adolescence but can occur at any age, comes from an autoimmune reaction that leads to the death of insulin-producing beta cells in the pancreas. As a result, persons with Type 1 Diabetes have an absolute lack of insulin, the hormone crucial for regulating blood sugar levels.

The management of Type 1 Diabetes relies on restoring the lost insulin with exogenous insulin therapy. This requires regular injections or the use of insulin pumps to imitate the body's natural insulin production. The purpose of insulin therapy is to maintain blood sugar levels within a specific range to prevent both short-term consequences, such as hypoglycemia (low blood sugar), and long-term complications, such as cardiovascular disease and nerve damage.

Monitoring blood sugar levels is an important element of controlling Type 1 Diabetes. Regular self-monitoring of blood glucose levels using a glucometer helps individuals make informed decisions about insulin dosing, food, and physical activity. Continuous glucose monitoring (CGM) systems deliver real-time data on blood sugar levels, providing useful insights into patterns and trends that might drive therapy adjustments.

In addition to insulin medication and blood sugar monitoring, patients with Type 1 Diabetes must also carefully regulate their food and exercise program. A balanced diet that includes whole grains, lean meats, fruits, vegetables, and healthy fats will help regulate blood sugar levels and enhance general health. Regular physical activity is also crucial for managing weight, maintaining insulin sensitivity, and reducing the risk of cardiovascular problems.

Beyond the physical components of controlling Type 1 Diabetes, it is necessary to address the emotional and psychological burden of living with a chronic disease. Coping with the demands of daily insulin therapy, blood sugar monitoring, and dietary restrictions can be tough, and support from healthcare providers, family, and peers can make a major difference in an individual's well-being.

Managing Type 1 Diabetes involves a multimodal approach that encompasses insulin administration, blood sugar monitoring, nutritional management, physical activity, and emotional support. By understanding the unique challenges associated with Type 1 Diabetes and adopting a complete management plan, individuals with this illness can enjoy full and healthy lives.

Pathophysiology of Type 1 Diabetes

Understanding the pathophysiology of Type 1 Diabetes provides essential insights into the underlying mechanisms driving this autoimmune illness. Type 1 Diabetes is defined by the loss of insulin-producing beta cells in the pancreas, leading to an absolute lack of insulin. This destruction is triggered by an autoimmune response when the body's immune system mistakenly labels beta cells as foreign invaders and mounts an attack against them.

The specific etiology of this autoimmune response in Type 1 Diabetes is not entirely understood, but genetic predisposition and environmental variables are considered to play significant roles. Certain genetic variations, notably within the human leukocyte antigen (HLA) complex, enhance the likelihood of acquiring Type 1 Diabetes. Environmental variables, such as virus infections, nutritional issues, and exposure to chemicals, may initiate or accelerate the autoimmune response in genetically vulnerable individuals.

The autoimmune attack on beta cells involves the activation of numerous immune cells, including T lymphocytes and macrophages, which infiltrate the pancreatic islets (clusters of cells in the pancreas) where beta cells are found. These immune cells emit pro-inflammatory cytokines and other signaling chemicals that cause inflammation and apoptosis (cell death) of beta cells.

As beta cell degeneration advances, insulin production falls, resulting in hyperglycemia (high blood sugar levels) and the hallmark symptoms of Type 1 Diabetes, such as excessive thirst, frequent urination, weight loss, and weariness. Without sufficient insulin, glucose cannot enter cells to give energy, resulting in metabolic imbalances and the creation of ketones as a consequence of fat breakdown, leading to a potentially life-threatening condition known as diabetic ketoacidosis (DKA).

In addition to the loss of beta cells, Type 1 Diabetes is accompanied by abnormalities in the balance of other pancreatic hormones, such as glucagon and somatostatin, which further contribute to dysregulation of blood sugar levels. Glucagon, produced by alpha cells in the pancreas, inhibits the action of insulin by increasing the release of glucose from the liver into the bloodstream, aggravating hyperglycemia in persons with Type 1 Diabetes.

The pathogenesis of Type 1 Diabetes is defined by an autoimmune attack on insulin-producing beta cells in the pancreas, resulting in an absolute lack of insulin and dysregulation of blood sugar levels. Genetic predisposition and environmental variables contribute to the development of an autoimmune response, resulting in the clinical signs of Type 1 Diabetes and its associated consequence

Diagnosis and Screening Techniques

Diagnosing and screening for diabetes requires a combination of clinical evaluation, laboratory tests, and assessment of risk factors to identify persons who may have the condition or be at risk of getting it. The technique is critical for early detection and intervention, which can help prevent or delay the onset of problems linked with diabetes.

One of the basic diagnostic tests for diabetes is the monitoring of blood glucose levels. The fasting plasma glucose (FPG) test, which involves evaluating blood sugar levels following an overnight fast, is often used to detect diabetes. A fasting blood glucose level of 126 milligrams per deciliter (mg/dL) or greater on two different occasions is indicative of diabetes.

Another diagnostic test is the oral glucose tolerance test (OGTT), which analyzes blood sugar levels before and two hours after drinking a glucose-rich beverage. A blood glucose level of 200 mg/dL or greater two hours after the glucose challenge validates the diagnosis of diabetes. The OGTT is very beneficial in identifying gestational diabetes during pregnancy.

The hemoglobin A1c (HbA1c) test is a measure of average blood glucose levels over the past two to three months and is used to assess long-term blood sugar control in persons with diabetes. A HbA1c result of 6.5% or greater is symptomatic of diabetes.

In addition to these diagnostic tests, screening for diabetes is indicated for persons with risk factors, such as obesity, family history of diabetes, history of gestational diabetes, and certain ethnic origins. Screening testing may include random blood glucose tests, HbA1c tests, and oral glucose tolerance tests, based on individual risk factors and clinical discretion.

Regular screening for diabetes is critical for early identification and intervention, as it enables healthcare practitioners to identify patients at risk of developing diabetes and undertake appropriate interventions to prevent or postpone its occurrence. Early detection and care can assist persons with diabetes achieve better blood sugar control and lower the risk of complications, such as cardiovascular disease, neuropathy, nephropathy, and retinopathy.

Diagnosing and screening for diabetes requires a combination of clinical evaluation, laboratory tests, and assessment of risk factors to identify persons who may have the condition or be at risk of getting it. Early detection and intervention are critical for preventing or delaying the onset of problems associated with diabetes, thereby improving health outcomes for persons living with the condition.

Evidence-Based Treatment Approaches

When it comes to treating diabetes, evidence-based treatments form the cornerstone of effective management. These techniques are rooted in rigorous scientific research and clinical trials, ensuring that therapies are based on solid evidence of their effectiveness in improving outcomes for individuals with diabetes.

One of the mainstays of evidence-based treatment for diabetes is lifestyle change. This involves dietary adjustments, frequent physical activity, weight management, and smoking cessation. Numerous studies have established the usefulness of lifestyle therapies in improving blood sugar control, reducing the risk of cardiovascular problems, and promoting general well-being for patients with diabetes.

Dietary management plays a significant part in diabetes therapy, with a focus on maintaining a balanced diet that is rich in fruits, vegetables, whole grains, lean proteins, and healthy fats. Carbohydrate counting and glycemic index considerations are regularly used ways to help patients with diabetes regulate their blood sugar levels efficiently.

Physical activity is another crucial component of evidence-based treatment for diabetes. Regular exercise increases insulin sensitivity, aids with weight management, and reduces the risk of cardiovascular disease. Both aerobic activity (such as walking, cycling, or swimming) and resistance training (such as weightlifting or resistance band exercises) have been demonstrated to be beneficial for those with diabetes.

Medication management is also a crucial element of evidence-based treatment for diabetes. For persons with Type 1 Diabetes, insulin therapy is necessary to replace the insulin that the body is unable to make. Various forms of insulin, including rapid-acting, short-acting, intermediate-acting, and long-acting formulations, are available to match individual needs and preferences.

For persons with Type 2 Diabetes, oral medicines, and injectable therapy may be administered to help improve blood sugar management. These drugs function by diverse means, such as enhancing insulin sensitivity, raising insulin production, decreasing glucose absorption in the intestines, or reducing glucose synthesis in the liver.

In addition to lifestyle adjustments and medication management, continuous monitoring of blood sugar levels and other pertinent indicators, such as blood pressure and cholesterol levels, is essential for efficient diabetes management. This allows healthcare providers to change treatment strategies as needed and identify any issues early.

Evidence-based treatment options for diabetes comprise lifestyle adjustments, medication management, and routine monitoring to achieve optimal blood sugar control and limit the risk of complications. By following evidence-based guidelines and working together with healthcare experts, individuals with diabetes can make proactive efforts to control their condition and improve their quality of life.

1.Insulin Therapy

Insulin therapy is an essential component of treatment for people who have type 1 diabetes, and it is also frequently utilized in the management of patients who have type 2 diabetes. A hormone that is produced by the pancreas, is responsible for regulating blood sugar levels. It does this by facilitating the uptake of glucose into cells, which is necessary for the creation of energy. In people who have diabetes, either the pancreas does not produce enough insulin (type 1 diabetes) or the cells in the body do not respond adequately to insulin (type 2 diabetes), which results in elevated blood sugar levels. Both types of diabetes ultimately lead to heart disease.

Exogenous insulin is administered through injections or insulin pumps in the course of insulin therapy, to imitate the natural insulin synthesis that occurs within the body. Based on their onset, peak, and duration of action, the various forms of insulin that are accessible can be organized into several categories. In a few minutes, rapid-acting insulin starts to function, reaches its peak between thirty minutes and three hours, and continues to work for three to five hours. Short-acting insulin begins to function within thirty minutes, reaches its peak between two and four hours, and continues to work for six to eight hours. Intermediate-acting insulin begins to exert its effects within two to four hours, reaches its peak within four to twelve hours, and continues to exert its effects for twelve to eighteen hours. The effects of long-acting insulin start to take effect within one to two hours, there is no noticeable peak, and it can last for up to twenty-four hours.

Personal characteristics, including as blood sugar levels, lifestyle choices, and treatment objectives, all play a role in determining which insulin regimen is most appropriate. Some individuals may require a basal-bolus regimen, which combines a mix of long-acting (basal) insulin to give background insulin coverage and rapid-acting (bolus) insulin to cover meals and correct high blood sugar levels. Others may utilize a premixed insulin regimen, which mixes a fixed combination of rapid-acting and intermediate-acting insulin in a single injection.

Insulin therapy demands regular monitoring of blood sugar levels to modify insulin doses as needed. Healthcare experts may advocate self-monitoring of blood glucose using a glucometer or continuous glucose monitoring (CGM) devices to measure blood sugar levels throughout the day. Regular follow-up visits with healthcare experts are crucial to examine blood sugar records, assess insulin doses, and address any concerns or questions about insulin therapy.

In addition to injections, insulin therapy can also be given by insulin pumps, which constantly infuse rapid-acting insulin beneath the skin through a tiny catheter. Insulin pumps give greater flexibility in insulin dose and mealtime insulin modifications and may be preferred by some patients, notably those with Type 1 Diabetes who require precise insulin delivery to meet their insulin needs.

Insulin therapy is a critical component of diabetes management for persons with Type 1 and Type 2 Diabetes. By delivering exogenous insulin to modulate blood sugar levels, insulin therapy helps individuals achieve improved glycemic control and lower the risk of diabetes-related complications. With proper education, monitoring, and assistance from healthcare experts, individuals can successfully incorporate insulin therapy into their daily lives and achieve optimal health results.

2. Continuous Glucose Monitoring (CGM)

Continuous Glucose Monitoring (CGM) has changed the management of diabetes by delivering real-time information regarding blood sugar levels throughout the day and night. This device comprises a tiny sensor implanted beneath the skin that detects glucose levels in the interstitial fluid, generally on the belly or upper arm. The sensor is attached to a transmitter that wirelessly feeds data to a receiver or smartphone app, allowing patients with diabetes and their healthcare practitioners to monitor blood sugar levels continually.

One of the primary benefits of CGM is its ability to provide real-time input on blood sugar levels, allowing individuals to make quick adjustments to their insulin doses, food, and physical activity. This proactive approach to diabetes treatment helps prevent hyperglycemia (high blood sugar) and hypoglycemia (low blood sugar) episodes, resulting in better overall blood sugar control and minimizing the risk of diabetes-related complications.

CGM also delivers insights into blood sugar patterns and trends over time, allowing patients and healthcare providers to spot patterns of hyperglycemia and hypoglycemia and make informed adjustments to treatment programs. By evaluating CGM data, healthcare clinicians can modify insulin regimens, nutritional suggestions, and lifestyle interventions to match individual needs and enhance glycemic control.

Moreover, CGM can assist people with diabetes in better understanding the impact of numerous factors, such as food choices, physical exercise, stress, and medication, on their blood sugar levels. This knowledge helps patients make informed decisions regarding their diabetes treatment and make proactive efforts to maintain optimal blood sugar control.

In addition to real-time monitoring, many CGM systems offer features such as alarms and notifications for high and low blood sugar levels, trend arrows indicating the direction and pace of blood sugar changes, and interaction with insulin pumps for automatic insulin delivery. These features enhance the usability and effectiveness of CGM systems, making them valuable tools for individuals with diabetes and their healthcare professionals.

Overall, Continuous Glucose Monitoring (CGM) has altered diabetes management by offering real-time insights about blood sugar levels and trends, empowering persons with diabetes to make informed decisions regarding their treatment and lifestyle. By exploiting the benefits of CGM technology, individuals can achieve improved glycemic control, minimize the risk of diabetes-related complications, and improve their quality of life.

3. Artificial Pancreas Systems

Artificial pancreas systems represent a significant advancement in diabetes care, offering a dynamic and automated approach to blood sugar management. These systems, also known as closed-loop systems, aim to mimic the function of a healthy pancreas by continually monitoring blood glucose levels and altering insulin supply in real-time.

Comprising an insulin pump and a continuous glucose monitor (CGM), an artificial pancreas system runs on sophisticated algorithms that understand the CGM data and automatically change insulin administration rates. This level of automation minimizes the load on patients with diabetes, giving a more seamless and precise technique to keep blood sugar levels within the therapeutic range.

One of the primary advantages of artificial pancreatic systems is their ability to respond promptly to variations in blood sugar levels. By constantly evaluating CGM data, the system can identify patterns and make prompt modifications to insulin delivery, preventing both hyperglycemia and hypoglycemia. This dynamic response is particularly advantageous at mealtime, exercise, and nighttime, addressing the issues that standard insulin delivery techniques may confront.

Individuals utilizing artificial pancreas devices frequently have improved blood sugar control, fewer hypoglycemia episodes, and enhanced overall quality of life. The automation of insulin delivery not only reduces the cognitive load associated with diabetes management but also provides for a more flexible lifestyle, permitting individuals to engage in regular activities with more confidence.

Despite these developments, it's crucial to highlight that artificial pancreatic systems are not a cure for diabetes. They serve as a significant tool in the management arsenal, necessitating continual collaboration between individuals with diabetes and their healthcare professionals. Regular monitoring, calibration, and tweaks to settings are important to ensure the system fits with individual needs and preferences.

As technology continues to progress, artificial pancreatic devices hold the potential for further modifications and enhancements. Research and development in this sector strive to improve the adaptability, user-friendliness, and accessibility of these systems, promoting a future where individuals with diabetes can have even greater autonomy and precision in their blood sugar management.

Lifestyle Modifications for Type 1 Diabetes Management

When it comes to controlling Type 1 Diabetes, lifestyle adjustments play a key part in achieving optimal blood sugar management and general well-being. Two major components of lifestyle adjustments for Type 1 Diabetes control include diet and nutrition, as well as exercise and physical activity.

Diet and Nutrition: Maintaining a balanced and nutritious diet is vital for those with Type 1 Diabetes to manage blood sugar levels efficiently. The cornerstone of a balanced diet for diabetes control includes consuming a variety of nutrient-rich foods, such as fruits, vegetables, whole grains, lean meats, and healthy fats. Emphasizing foods with a low glycemic index will help prevent blood sugar rises and encourage consistent energy levels throughout the day.

Carbohydrate counting is a great tool for patients with Type 1 Diabetes to regulate their blood sugar levels. Since carbs have the most important impact on blood sugar, monitoring carbohydrate consumption and changing insulin doses accordingly can help maintain optimal blood sugar management. Working with a licensed dietitian or diabetes educator can provide direction and help in implementing carbohydrate counting and meal planning strategies adapted to individual requirements and preferences.

In addition to carbohydrate counting, portion control, and mindful eating are critical parts of treating Type 1 Diabetes. Monitoring portion sizes and paying attention to hunger and fullness cues can help prevent overeating and promote improved blood sugar regulation. It's also vital to minimize the intake of sugary and processed meals, as these might cause rapid rises in blood sugar levels.

Exercise and Physical Activity: Regular exercise and physical activity are beneficial for individuals with Type 1 Diabetes in various ways. Physical activity can enhance insulin sensitivity, allowing the body to use insulin more efficiently to lower blood sugar levels. It also helps weight management, reduces cardiovascular risk factors, and enhances general health and well-being.

Incorporating a variety of physical activities into everyday life, such as brisk walking, cycling, swimming, weight training, and yoga, can assist individuals with Type 1 Diabetes reach their fitness objectives and maintaining optimal blood sugar control. It's crucial to find activities that are pleasurable and sustainable to encourage long-term adherence.

Before starting any exercise program, individuals with Type 1 Diabetes should check with their healthcare professional to ensure that their exercise plan is safe and appropriate for their unique health condition and needs. Monitoring blood sugar levels before, during, and after exercise, and making modifications to insulin dosages or carbohydrate consumption as appropriate, can help prevent hypoglycemia (low blood sugar) and enhance performance and recovery.

Lifestyle adjustments, including diet and nutrition, as well as exercise and physical activity, are critical components of controlling Type 1 Diabetes effectively. By adopting healthy dietary habits, managing carbohydrate intake, and engaging in regular physical activity, individuals with Type 1 Diabetes can achieve better blood sugar control, lower the risk of complications, and develop their total quality of life.

Psychosocial Considerations and Support for Type 1 Diabetes Patients

Psychosocial considerations and support are key parts of managing Type 1 diabetes, as they address the emotional and psychological burden of living with a chronic illness. Dealing with the daily obstacles of diabetes care, such as blood sugar monitoring, insulin injections, dietary restrictions, and potential consequences, can take a toll on an individual's emotional well-being. Therefore, it's crucial to recognize and manage the psychosocial elements of type 1 diabetes to ensure comprehensive care for patients.

One of the main psychosocial considerations for patients with type 1 Diabetes is the emotional impact of the diagnosis. Being diagnosed with a chronic disease can trigger a range of feelings, including fear, anger, despair, and worry. It's typical for individuals to suffer sentiments of sadness and loss for their pre-diagnosis lifestyle and anxiety about the future implications of diabetes. Providing emotional support and validation for these sentiments is vital in helping patients navigate their emotional journey with diabetes.

In addition to emotional support, practical help and knowledge are also vital for those with Type 1 Diabetes. Learning to manage diabetes effectively entails acquiring new skills and knowledge about blood sugar monitoring, insulin delivery, carbohydrate counting, and recognizing and responding to hypoglycemia and hyperglycemia. Education classes, workshops, and support groups can give vital knowledge and resources to empower people in their diabetes care journey.

Family and social support also play a crucial role in assisting patients with type 1 diabetes. Family members and close friends can provide emotional support, encouragement, and practical assistance with diabetes care activities. Involving family members in diabetes education sessions and treatment planning can establish a supportive and collaborative environment that supports improved diabetes management outcomes.

Psychosocial care for Type 1 diabetes patients also extends to treating concerns linked to self-esteem, body image, and social interactions. Living with a visible medical condition like diabetes can sometimes lead to feelings of self-consciousness, stigma, and social isolation. Encouraging open communication, giving chances for peer support, and encouraging positive self-image and self-acceptance can assist individuals with type 1 diabetes in negotiating social problems with confidence and resilience.

Furthermore, addressing mental health concerns, such as depression, anxiety, and diabetic distress, is vital to providing comprehensive care for patients with type 1 diabetes. Mental health screening, access to counseling services, and referrals to mental health specialists can help people manage their emotional well-being and cope more effectively with the challenges of living with diabetes.

Psychosocial concerns and support are key components of managing type 1 diabetes effectively. By addressing the emotional, practical, social, and mental health elements of living with diabetes, healthcare practitioners can provide holistic care that improves overall well-being and allows patients to live happy lives despite their chronic diseases.

Chapter 2

Type 2 Diabetes: Pathogenesis and Intervention Strategies

Understanding the pathophysiology of type 2 diabetes is critical to developing effective intervention techniques to control and prevent this chronic condition. Type 2 diabetes develops when the body grows resistant to the effects of insulin or when the pancreas fails to generate enough insulin to meet the body's needs. Insulin resistance occurs when cells in the body, notably muscle, fat, and liver cells, do not respond adequately to insulin and fail to take up glucose from the bloodstream, resulting in high blood sugar levels.

Several factors contribute to the development of insulin resistance in type 2 diabetes, including genetic predisposition, obesity, a sedentary lifestyle, and dietary choices. Genetic factors can alter insulin sensitivity and insulin production, increasing the likelihood of developing type 2 diabetes. Obesity, particularly excess visceral fat (fat stored around the belly), is highly connected with insulin resistance, as adipose tissue emits inflammatory cytokines and hormones that impede insulin signaling.

Physical inactivity and a sedentary lifestyle also lead to insulin resistance and the development of type 2 diabetes. Regular physical activity increases insulin sensitivity, enhances glucose uptake by muscles, and helps maintain a healthy weight, minimizing the incidence of insulin resistance and type 2 diabetes. Conversely, a sedentary lifestyle and lack of exercise can aggravate insulin resistance and raise the chance of acquiring type 2 diabetes.

Dietary variables also play a crucial influence in the etiology of Type 2 Diabetes. Consuming a diet high in refined carbs, sugars, and saturated fats can contribute to insulin resistance, obesity, and raised blood sugar levels. Conversely, a diet rich in whole grains, fruits, vegetables, lean meats, and healthy fats can increase insulin sensitivity, promote weight loss, and minimize the risk of Type 2 Diabetes.

Intervention options for managing and preventing Type 2 diabetes focus on reducing insulin resistance, promoting weight loss, and improving overall metabolic health. Lifestyle alterations, including dietary changes, frequent physical activity, and weight management, are the foundation of Type 2 diabetes therapy. Adopting a balanced diet that emphasizes whole foods, portion control, and nutrient-dense selections will help improve insulin sensitivity and blood sugar control.

Regular physical activity, including aerobic exercise and resistance training, is vital for improving insulin sensitivity, facilitating weight loss, and reducing the risk of type 2 diabetes. Objective for at least 150 minutes of moderate-intensity aerobic activity or 75 minutes of vigorous-intensity aerobic activity per week, sideways with muscle-strengthening activities on two or more days per week.

In addition to lifestyle improvements, pharmaceutical therapies may be indicated for people with type 2 diabetes who do not achieve glycemic objectives through lifestyle changes alone. Oral medicines, such as metformin, sulfonylureas, thiazolidinediones, DPP-4 inhibitors, SGLT2 inhibitors, and GLP-1 receptor agonists, are often used to improve blood sugar control and minimize the risk of diabetes-related complications.

Type 2 diabetes develops owing to insulin resistance and decreased insulin production, impacted by genetic, lifestyle, and nutritional variables. Intervention options for managing and preventing Type 2 diabetes focus on addressing insulin resistance, promoting weight loss, and improving metabolic health through lifestyle modifications and, if necessary, pharmaceutical therapies. By adopting a healthy lifestyle and working closely with healthcare experts, individuals with type 2 diabetes can achieve better blood sugar management and lower the risk of complications associated with this chronic condition.

Mechanisms Underlying Type 2 Diabetes Development

Understanding the mechanisms behind the development of Type 2 Diabetes is vital for unraveling the intricacies of this chronic condition. Type 2 Diabetes develops when the body grows resistant to the effects of insulin or when the pancreas fails to generate enough insulin to meet the body's needs. Insulin resistance is a crucial element in the pathophysiology of Type 2 Diabetes, defined by impaired responsiveness of cells, notably in muscle, fat, and liver tissues, to the action of insulin. As a result, these cells are less able to take up glucose from the bloodstream, leading to higher blood sugar levels.

Several factors contribute to the development of insulin resistance in Type 2 Diabetes, including genetic predisposition, obesity, sedentary lifestyle, and dietary choices. Genetic factors can alter insulin sensitivity and insulin production, increasing the likelihood of developing Type 2 Diabetes. Obesity, particularly excess visceral fat (fat stored around the belly), is highly connected with insulin resistance, as adipose tissue emits inflammatory cytokines and hormones that impede insulin signaling.

In addition to genetics and obesity, lifestyle variables such as physical inactivity and poor eating habits also play a key role in the development of insulin resistance and Type 2 Diabetes. Regular physical activity increases insulin sensitivity, enhances glucose uptake by muscles, and helps maintain a healthy weight, minimizing the incidence of insulin resistance and Type 2 Diabetes. Conversely, a sedentary lifestyle and lack of exercise can aggravate insulin resistance and raise the chance of acquiring Type 2 Diabetes.

Dietary variables also contribute to the development of Type 2 Diabetes. Consuming a diet high in refined carbs, sugars, and saturated fats can contribute to insulin resistance, obesity, and raised blood sugar levels. Conversely, a diet rich in whole grains, fruits, vegetables, lean meats, and healthy fats can increase insulin sensitivity, promote weight loss, and minimize the risk of Type 2 Diabetes.

The mechanisms underlying the development of Type 2 Diabetes involve a complex combination of genetic, lifestyle, and nutritional factors. Insulin resistance, driven by genetic predisposition, obesity, physical inactivity, and poor dietary habits, plays a crucial role in the etiology of Type 2 Diabetes. By knowing these pathways, healthcare providers can develop focused therapies to prevent and manage Type 2 Diabetes effectively, focusing on lifestyle adjustments, weight control, and improving insulin sensitivity.

Diagnostic Criteria and Screening Recommendations

Understanding the diagnostic criteria and screening recommendations for Type 2 Diabetes is critical for early detection and efficient management of this chronic condition. The diagnosis criteria for Type 2 Diabetes are based on blood sugar levels obtained by particular laboratory testing. The American Diabetes Association (ADA) recommends utilizing one of the following tests to identify Type 2 Diabetes: fasting plasma glucose (FPG) test, oral glucose tolerance test (OGTT), or hemoglobin A1c (HbA1c) test.

The fasting plasma glucose (FPG) test measures blood sugar levels after an overnight fast of at least 8 hours. A blood sugar level of 126 milligrams per deciliter (mg/dL) or greater on two different occasions suggests Type 2 Diabetes. The oral glucose tolerance test (OGTT) involves drinking a sweet solution and monitoring blood sugar levels before and 2 hours after ingestion. A blood sugar level of 200 mg/dL or greater after 2 hours validates the diagnosis of Type 2 Diabetes.

The hemoglobin A1c (HbA1c) test evaluates the average blood sugar levels over the last 2-3 months by determining the proportion of hemoglobin that is glycated (bound to glucose). An HbA1c reading of 6.5% or higher suggests Type 2 Diabetes. It's vital to highlight that the diagnosis of Type 2 Diabetes should be confirmed with a repeat test on a separate day, using the same test procedure, to rule out laboratory error or transitory hyperglycemia.

In addition to diagnostic testing, screening strategies for Type 2 Diabetes attempt to identify those at risk of developing the condition before symptoms show. The ADA recommends screening for Type 2 Diabetes in asymptomatic adults who are overweight or obese (body mass index ≥ 25 kg/m²) and have one or more additional risk factors, including family history of diabetes, sedentary lifestyle, high blood pressure, dyslipidemia (abnormal blood lipid levels), or history of gestational diabetes or polycystic ovary syndrome (PCOS).

The optimal screening test for Type 2 Diabetes in asymptomatic adults is the fasting plasma glucose

(FPG) test or the hemoglobin A1c (HbA1c) test. These tests are easy, cost-effective, and have good sensitivity and specificity for identifying diabetes. The ADA recommends repeating screening tests every 3 years in persons with normal findings, and more frequently in those with prediabetes or other risk factors.

Understanding the diagnostic criteria and screening recommendations for Type 2 Diabetes is critical for early detection and efficient management of this chronic condition. Diagnostic procedures such as the fasting plasma glucose (FPG) test, oral glucose tolerance test (OGTT), and hemoglobin A1c (HbA1c) test can confirm the diagnosis of Type 2 Diabetes while screening recommendations try to identify persons at risk before symptoms occur. By instituting regular screening and diagnostic tests, healthcare practitioners can identify and intervene early in persons with Type 2 Diabetes, leading to better outcomes and improved quality of life.

Pharmacological Interventions for Type 2 Diabetes

Pharmacological therapies for Type 2 Diabetes have advanced dramatically, enabling a varied array of alternatives to maintain blood sugar levels efficiently. These approaches largely fall into three categories: oral antidiabetic medicines, injectable therapies, and new pharmacotherapies with promising future possibilities.

Oral Antidiabetic Medications:

Oral antidiabetic medicines are available in various classes, each targeting different parts of glucose metabolism to assist in lowering blood sugar levels. Metformin, the cornerstone of oral treatment, acts by lowering glucose synthesis in the liver and enhancing insulin sensitivity in peripheral tissues. Sulfonylureas and meglitinides promote insulin release from the pancreas, while thiazolidinediones enhance insulin sensitivity in muscle and fat cells. DPP-4 inhibitors and SGLT2 inhibitors function on distinct mechanisms to reduce blood sugar levels by inhibiting the breakdown of incretin hormones and promoting urine glucose excretion, respectively. Alpha-glucosidase inhibitors slow down carbohydrate digestion and absorption in the intestines, hence lowering postprandial blood sugar rises.

Injectable Therapies: Injectable therapies are designated for persons with Type 2 Diabetes who do not maintain acceptable blood sugar control with oral drugs alone. Insulin therapy remains the most effective treatment for reducing blood sugar levels in Type 2 Diabetes by replacing or boosting the body's insulin production. Different types of insulin formulations, including rapid-acting, short-acting, intermediate-acting, and long-acting insulin, are available to replicate the body's natural insulin secretion patterns. Glucagon-like peptide-1 receptor agonist (GLP-1 RAs) are injectable drugs that boost insulin production, decrease glucagon release, slow gastric emptying, and enhance satiety, leading to improved blood sugar control and weight loss.

Emerging Pharmacotherapies and Future Directions: The field of Type 2 Diabetes care is witnessing significant breakthroughs in pharmacotherapy with the discovery of innovative medicines and treatment techniques. Dual and triple therapy combinations, combining drugs from various classes with complementary mechanisms of action, give synergistic effects and enhanced glycemic control. Beyond typical pharmacological targets, researchers are exploring new ways, such as targeting gut hormone receptors and altering gut microbiota, to regulate glucose metabolism and promote metabolic health. Additionally, personalized medicine approaches, integrating genetic and molecular analysis, hold promise for adapting treatments to individual patient features and maximizing therapeutic outcomes.

Pharmaceutical therapies into a comprehensive treatment plan for Type 2 Diabetes involves a multidisciplinary approach comprising healthcare practitioners, including primary care physicians, endocrinologists, diabetes educators, and pharmacists. Regular monitoring of blood sugar levels, drug adherence, and potential adverse effects is required to ensure maximum efficacy and safety of pharmacotherapy. By staying current on ongoing research and improvements in pharmacotherapies, healthcare providers can continue to strengthen the management of Type 2 Diabetes and improve patient outcomes.

Lifestyle Interventions for Type 2 Diabetes Management

Effectively managing Type 2 Diabetes goes beyond drugs; lifestyle modifications play a crucial role in achieving and maintaining optimal blood sugar control. Let's analyze the essential components of lifestyle interventions: food approaches, exercise routines, and weight management measures.

Dietary Approaches: A well-balanced and attentive approach to eating is important in managing Type 2 Diabetes. Emphasizing entire, nutrient-dense foods can have a tremendous impact on blood sugar levels. Prioritizing fiber-rich foods such as fruits, vegetables, whole grains, and legumes helps manage blood sugar by slowing down digestion and absorption. Carbohydrate counting, recognizing portion proportions, and spacing meals throughout the day can lead to more stable blood sugar levels. Additionally, consuming lean proteins, and healthy fats, and minimizing processed and sugary foods can further promote general metabolic health.

Exercise Regimens: Physical activity is a cornerstone in the management of Type 2 Diabetes, delivering a plethora of advantages. Regular exercise enhances insulin sensitivity, allowing cells to more efficiently utilize glucose. Both aerobic workouts, such as brisk walking, swimming, or cycling, and resistance training, which includes sports like weightlifting, lead to better blood sugar control. The American Diabetes Association recommends at least 150 minutes of moderate-intensity aerobic activity each week, along with muscle-strengthening exercises at least two days per week. Tailoring workout programs to individual interests and capabilities ensures sustainability and enjoyment.

Weight Management Strategies: Maintaining a healthy weight is closely linked to improved blood sugar management in Type 2 Diabetes. Even minor weight loss can have major benefits. Adopting a holistic approach that incorporates food adjustments and increased physical activity is successful in achieving and sustaining weight loss. Setting realistic objectives, focusing on gradual improvements, and obtaining advice from healthcare professionals or dietitians can enhance the success of weight management measures. Beyond the numbers on the scale, the distribution of body fat, particularly visceral fat around the abdomen, is crucial, as it is connected with insulin resistance.

Integrating these lifestyle modifications throughout daily life demands dedication and consistency. Creating a supportive environment that includes family, friends, and healthcare providers can dramatically improve adherence to these adjustments. Regular monitoring of blood sugar levels and adjustments to lifestyle measures based on individual responses are needed to adapt management methods effectively.

Lifestyle therapies are crucial to the complete management of Type 2 Diabetes. Dietary methods, exercise regimes, and weight management measures comprise a dynamic trinity that empowers individuals to take an active role in their health. By accepting these lifestyle adjustments, individuals with Type 2 Diabetes can maximize their blood sugar control, increase overall well-being, and establish a sustainable basis for long-term health.

Chapter 3

Beyond Type 1 and Type 2: Other Forms of Diabetes

Beyond Type 1 and Type 2 Diabetes, there exist other kinds of diabetes that are less frequent but equally important to diagnose and understand. These variants may have distinct causes, processes, and management considerations, highlighting the heterogeneous character of diabetes.

One of these is gestational diabetes, which arises during pregnancy and normally resolves after childbirth. Gestational diabetes develops when the body cannot create enough insulin to satisfy the increasing demands of pregnancy, leading to raised blood sugar levels. While gestational diabetes frequently recovers postpartum, it raises the chance of acquiring Type 2 Diabetes later in life for both the mother and the child. Managing gestational diabetes entails dietary adjustments, monitoring blood sugar levels, and sometimes insulin therapy to achieve optimal mother and fetal health during pregnancy.

Another form of diabetes is monogenic diabetes, which originates from mutations in a single gene that alters insulin synthesis or activity. Monogenic diabetes is rare and can develop in childhood or maturity, mimicking signs of both Type 1 and Type 2 Diabetes. Identifying the specific genetic mutation responsible for monogenic diabetes is critical for individualized treatment methods. Management may require oral medicines, insulin therapy, or other specific interventions based on the underlying genetic abnormality.

Cystic fibrosis-related diabetes (CFRD) is another distinct kind of diabetes that affects persons with cystic fibrosis, a genetic condition that primarily affects the lungs and digestive system. CFRD occurs owing to pancreatic injury and decreased insulin production, leading to glucose intolerance and diabetes. Managing CFRD involves a multidisciplinary approach, including enhancing lung function, nutritional support, and insulin therapy to maintain stable blood sugar levels and prevent complications.

Additionally, steroid-induced diabetes is a form of diabetes that occurs as a side effect of long-term steroid therapy for illnesses such as autoimmune disorders, asthma, or organ donation. Steroids can reduce insulin sensitivity and increase glucose synthesis, resulting in increased blood sugar levels. Managing steroid-induced diabetes entails closely monitoring blood sugar levels, reducing steroid doses if possible, and implementing lifestyle modifications and pharmacological therapy to control blood sugar levels efficiently.

Overall, understanding and recognizing these additional forms of diabetes is essential for accurate diagnosis and effective care. While Type 1 and Type 2 Diabetes are the most frequent kinds, embracing the varied spectrum of diabetes enables healthcare providers to personalize treatment strategies and support individuals with diabetes in reaching optimal health outcomes

Gestational Diabetes Mellitus (GDM)

Gestational Diabetes Mellitus (GDM) is a type of diabetes that develops during pregnancy and normally resolves after childbirth. However, it requires careful treatment to protect the health of both the mother and the infant. Let's review the screening and diagnosis process, as well as management alternatives for GDM.

Screening and Diagnosis: Screening for GDM typically occurs between 24 and 28 weeks of gestation, although it may be recommended earlier in high-risk individuals. The screening technique involves a glucose challenge test (GCT), when the pregnant lady drinks a sweet solution, followed by a blood draw to determine blood sugar levels. If the initial screening test is abnormal, a diagnostic glucose tolerance test (GTT) is performed to confirm the diagnosis. During the GTT, blood sugar levels are measured after fasting and at regular intervals following the ingestion of a glucose solution.

The diagnostic criteria for GDM vary by country and medical organization, but generally involve specific thresholds for fasting, one-hour, and two-hour blood sugar levels during the GTT. Diagnosis of GDM is based on these glucose readings meeting or above the defined limits. It's important to remember that early detection and diagnosis of GDM are crucial for adopting prompt therapies to manage blood sugar levels and prevent issues for both the mother and the baby.

Management Strategies: The management of GDM focuses on controlling blood sugar levels to minimize the risk of complications during pregnancy and delivery. Dietary adjustments, regular physical activity, and sometimes pharmacological therapy are critical components of GDM management.

Dietary management involves working with a registered dietitian to develop a personalized meal plan that emphasizes complex carbohydrates, fiber-rich foods, lean proteins, and healthy fats. Portion control, timing meals throughout the day, and monitoring carbohydrate intake are crucial measures for regulating blood sugar levels. Regular physical activity, such as walking or prenatal yoga, can also help improve insulin sensitivity and regulate blood sugar levels.

In rare circumstances, pharmaceutical therapy may be necessary to achieve optimal blood sugar control in GDM. Insulin is the most common medication used in GDM management, as it does not cross the placenta and is considered safe for the baby. Oral medications, such as metformin or glyburide, may be considered in certain situations under the guidance of a healthcare provider.

Additionally, frequent monitoring of blood sugar levels throughout pregnancy is necessary for changing management measures as needed. Regular prenatal appointments, including evaluating fetal growth and well-being, are particularly crucial to guarantee the health and safety of both the mother and the baby.

Screening, diagnosis, and management of GDM are critical parts of prenatal care to ensure the health and well-being of both the mother and the infant. Early detection through screening tests, followed by personalized management strategies involving dietary modifications, physical activity, and sometimes medication therapy, are key to achieving optimal blood sugar control and preventing complications associated with GDM. Working closely with a healthcare team, including obstetricians, endocrinologists, registered dietitians, and diabetes educators, can help ensure the best possible outcomes for pregnant individuals with GDM.

Monogenic Diabetes

Monogenic Diabetes is a rare form of diabetes that originates from mutations in a single gene, altering insulin synthesis or activity. Unlike Type 1 and Type 2 Diabetes, which are complex illnesses impacted by both hereditary and environmental factors, monogenic diabetes is caused by unique genetic mutations inherited from one or both parents.

Genetic Basis and Clinical Characteristics: Monogenic diabetes covers various subtypes, including maturity-onset diabetes of the young (MODY), neonatal diabetes mellitus (NDM), and congenital hyperinsulinism (CHI). Each subtype is defined by specific genetic alterations and clinical characteristics.

MODY, for example, is often diagnosed in youth or early adulthood and is sometimes misdiagnosed as Type 1 or Type 2 Diabetes. It is caused by abnormalities in genes important in beta-cell activity and insulin secretion, resulting in poor glucose regulation. NDM, on the other hand, manifests shortly after birth and is caused by mutations altering insulin synthesis or action.

CHI is a rare form of diabetes that develops in infancy and is characterized by increased insulin secretion due to abnormalities in genes encoding proteins involved in insulin secretion.

Diagnosis of monogenic diabetes involves genetic testing to identify specific mutations related to the illness. Clinical characteristics, family history, and age of onset are additional relevant variables in reaching a diagnosis. Unlike Type 1 and Type 2 Diabetes, which are commonly diagnosed primarily on clinical presentation and laboratory tests, the diagnosis of monogenic diabetes requires specialist genetic testing.

Treatment Approaches: Treatment of monogenic diabetes differs based on the precise subtype and genetic mutation involved. In general, management strives to maximize blood sugar control and prevent long-term problems associated with diabetes.

For persons with MODY, treatment may involve lifestyle modifications, like as dietary changes and regular physical activity, to control blood sugar levels. Some individuals may require oral drugs, such as sulfonylureas or insulin secretagogues, to stimulate insulin secretion and improve glycemic control.

Neonatal diabetes mellitus (NDM) and congenital hyperinsulinism (CHI) require more rigorous management, often involving insulin therapy or other drugs to regulate blood sugar levels. In some cases of NDM, individuals may switch from insulin therapy to sulfonylurea medicines, which can effectively maintain blood sugar levels by increasing insulin secretion.

Genetic counseling is an essential part of the therapy of monogenic diabetes since it provides people and families with knowledge of the underlying genetic etiology of the ailment, inheritance patterns, and implications for family members. Understanding the genetic basis of monogenic diabetes might assist guide treatment options and advise family planning.

Monogenic diabetes is a rare form of diabetes caused by particular genetic abnormalities altering insulin synthesis or activity. Diagnosis needs genetic testing and evaluation of clinical characteristics, age of onset, and family history. Treatment techniques differ according

to the subtype and genetic mutation implicated, with choices ranging from lifestyle adjustments to pharmacological therapy. hereditary counseling is vital for individuals and families afflicted by monogenic diabetes to understand the hereditary basis of the condition and make informed decisions regarding treatment and family planning. Despite its rarity, understanding monogenic diabetes is vital for healthcare practitioners to guarantee proper diagnosis and adequate therapy, thereby improving outcomes for persons with this condition.

Other Rare Forms of Diabetes

When it comes to diabetes, Maturity-Onset Diabetes of the Young (MODY) and Latent Autoimmune Diabetes in Adults (LADA) are two lesser-known but significant kinds that demand consideration.

Maturity-Onset Diabetes of the Young (MODY): MODY is a rare form of diabetes that often presents before the age of 25 and is defined by autosomal dominant inheritance, meaning it can be passed down through generations in families. Unlike Type 1 and Type 2 Diabetes, which are complex illnesses impacted by hereditary and environmental factors, MODY develops from mutations in specific genes involved in beta-cell activity and insulin secretion. These genetic abnormalities affect normal glucose homeostasis, resulting in high blood sugar levels and diabetic symptoms. MODY subtypes include mutations in genes such as HNF1A, HNF4A, and GCK, each with unique clinical manifestations and therapeutic considerations. Diagnosis of MODY entails genetic testing to identify specific mutations related to the disorder, as well as assessment of clinical characteristics and family history.

Latent Autoimmune Diabetes in Adults (LADA): LADA is a kind of diabetes that shares characteristics of both Type 1 and Type 2 Diabetes and is commonly referred to as "Type 1.5 Diabetes." LADA often manifests in adulthood, usually after the age of 30, and is defined by autoimmune death of pancreatic beta cells, similar to Type 1 Diabetes. However, unlike typical Type 1 Diabetes, which emerges in infancy or adolescence, LADA develops more gradually and initially may not require insulin therapy. Individuals with LADA often demonstrate autoimmune signs, such as the existence of autoantibodies against pancreatic beta cells, similar to those reported in Type 1 Diabetes. Diagnosis of LADA comprises clinical evaluation, antibody testing, and assessment of insulin secretion capacity. Management of LADA may require lifestyle adjustments, oral medicines, and eventually insulin therapy as beta-cell activity declines over time.

While MODY and LADA are less frequent than Type 1 and Type 2 Diabetes, they constitute major subgroups with distinct genetic and clinical features. Recognizing these unusual kinds of diabetes is critical for correct diagnosis and appropriate management, as they may require different treatment approaches compared to traditional Type 1 and Type 2 Diabetes. Further research and awareness of MODY and LADA are needed to better knowledge, diagnosis, and management of these specific forms of diabetes.

Challenges and Considerations in Managing Rare Forms of Diabetes

Managing unusual forms of diabetes, such as Maturity-Onset Diabetes of the Young (MODY), Latent Autoimmune Diabetes in Adults (LADA), and other less prevalent subtypes, poses distinct challenges and considerations for healthcare providers and persons afflicted by these disorders.

One of the main obstacles in managing unusual forms of diabetes is the poor understanding and acknowledgment of these illnesses among healthcare practitioners. Due to their rarity, unusual forms of diabetes may not be frequently evaluated in the differential diagnosis, leading to delayed or missed diagnoses. This can result in suboptimal management and potentially bad consequences for persons with these illnesses.

Furthermore, genetic testing for rare forms of diabetes, such as MODY, may not be readily available or accessible in all healthcare settings. Genetic testing is vital for diagnosing MODY and identifying particular genetic variants related to the disorder. However, the availability of genetic testing varies based on factors such as geographical location, healthcare resources, and insurance coverage, creating a barrier to rapid diagnosis and therapy.

Another problem is the lack of established treatment protocols for uncommon kinds of diabetes. Unlike Type 1 and Type 2 Diabetes, which have well-established treatment algorithms and management techniques, unusual forms of diabetes may require personalized therapies based on the exact subtype and genetic mutation involved. This tailored approach to therapy involves expertise in unusual forms of diabetes and may necessitate coordination with specialists such as endocrinologists and geneticists.

Additionally, managing unusual types of diabetes generally includes addressing unique clinical issues and comorbidities associated with these illnesses. For example, those with LADA may have autoimmune-related issues that require specialist care, whereas those with MODY may have challenges relating to familial inheritance patterns and genetic counseling.

Despite these limitations, breakthroughs in genetic testing, molecular diagnostics, and precision medicine offer great potential for improving the diagnosis and management of uncommon forms of diabetes.

Increased awareness among healthcare providers, enhanced access to genetic testing, and multidisciplinary teamwork are critical for addressing the special needs of persons with uncommon forms of diabetes and enhancing their long-term health outcomes.

Managing unusual forms of diabetes requires overcoming many hurdles, including limited awareness among healthcare providers, accessibility of genetic testing, and tailored treatment techniques. By addressing these issues and recognizing the particular clinical considerations associated with uncommon forms of diabetes, healthcare practitioners can improve the diagnosis and management of these illnesses and ultimately enhance the quality of care for patients afflicted by rare forms of diabetes.

Chapter 4

Integrative Approaches to Diabetes Management

Integrative approaches to diabetes care comprise a comprehensive approach that blends conventional medical treatments with complementary therapies and lifestyle adjustments. These integrative treatments try to address the multidimensional character of diabetes by treating not only blood sugar levels but also underlying variables such as inflammation, oxidative stress, and lifestyle factors.

One essential component of integrative diabetic care is dietary adjustment. Adopting a balanced and nutrient-rich diet can play a key role in regulating blood sugar levels and minimizing the risk of problems linked with diabetes. Emphasizing nutritious foods, such as fruits, vegetables, whole grains, and lean proteins, while reducing processed and sugary foods, can help manage blood sugar levels and support general health.

In addition to dietary adjustments, physical activity is another key part of integrative diabetes management. Regular exercise can improve insulin sensitivity, facilitate weight loss or weight management, and enhance cardiovascular health. Incorporating a variety of activities, such as aerobic exercise, weight training, and flexibility exercises, can give overall advantages to those with diabetes.

Complementary therapies, such as acupuncture, yoga, and mindfulness meditation, are increasingly gaining recognition for their potential advantages in diabetes control. These therapies can help reduce stress, enhance sleep quality, and boost general well-being, which are essential considerations in controlling diabetes and its related problems.

Furthermore, herbal supplements and botanical treatments are rapidly being examined for their possible significance in diabetes control. Certain herbs and supplements, including as cinnamon, fenugreek, and chromium, have been examined for their effects on blood sugar levels and insulin sensitivity. However, it's vital to approach these supplements with caution and contact a healthcare expert before incorporating them into a diabetic treatment strategy.

Integrative diabetes management also involves addressing mental and emotional well-being, as stress and psychological variables can affect blood sugar levels and general health. strategies such as cognitive-behavioral therapy (CBT), stress management strategies, and support groups can assist patients with diabetes cope with the emotional issues connected with their condition and enhance their quality of life.

Integrative approaches to diabetes care offer a complete and tailored approach that covers the different needs of persons with diabetes. By integrating conventional medical treatments with complementary therapies, lifestyle modifications, and psychological support, integrative diabetes management attempts to maximize blood sugar control, increase overall health, and enhance the well-being of those living with diabetes.

Holistic Care Models for Diabetes

Holistic care strategies for diabetes emphasize a comprehensive approach to managing the condition by addressing not just the physical components but also the emotional, social, and psychological factors that affect a person's health and well-being. These models emphasize that diabetes is a complicated and diverse disorder that demands a personalized and integrated approach to therapy.

One essential feature of holistic care approaches for diabetes is patient-centered care. This strategy entails actively integrating individuals with diabetes into their own care and treatment decisions, taking into consideration their preferences, values, and goals. By allowing patients to participate in their care, healthcare practitioners can better accommodate their specific needs and preferences, leading to improved health outcomes and patient satisfaction.

Another crucial component of holistic care models for diabetes is interdisciplinary collaboration. Diabetes management sometimes requires involvement from many healthcare specialists, including endocrinologists, primary care physicians, nutritionists, diabetes educators, psychologists, and social workers. By working together as a team, these experts can provide comprehensive and coordinated treatment that addresses the different requirements of patients with diabetes.

In addition to medical management, holistic care models for diabetes also emphasize lifestyle adjustments and self-management measures. This involves supporting good food choices, frequent physical activity, stress management skills, and medication adherence. By giving patients the knowledge and skills to manage their diabetes successfully, holistic care models can help improve their overall health and quality of life.

Furthermore, comprehensive care approaches for diabetes highlight the need to address social determinants of health and remove barriers to care. This may involve giving access to resources such as inexpensive nutritious food options, transportation help, and support services for mental health and social well-being. By addressing these social issues, healthcare providers can better help patients with diabetes in reaching optimal health outcomes.

Finally, holistic care approaches for diabetes highlight the significance of continual monitoring and follow-up treatment. Regular monitoring of blood sugar levels, medication adherence, and lifestyle choices is critical for identifying and treating any changes or issues in diabetes care. Follow-up consultations with healthcare experts allow for continuing assessment and revision of treatment plans as needed, ensuring that individuals with diabetes receive the support and assistance they need to properly manage their disease.

Holistic care methods for diabetes emphasize a holistic and integrated approach to managing the condition that covers the physical, emotional, social, and psychological components of health. By embracing patient-centered treatment, interdisciplinary teamwork, lifestyle adjustments, and addressing socioeconomic determinants of health, holistic care approaches can assist improve health outcomes and quality of life for those living with diabetes.

Integrating Traditional and Complementary Therapies

Integrating traditional and complementary therapies in healthcare, including diabetes management, is gaining recognition as a holistic strategy that addresses the various requirements of individuals and complements conventional medical treatments. Traditional therapies, including medicines and insulin therapy, are fundamental components of diabetes management and play a crucial role in managing blood sugar levels. However, alternative therapies, such as acupuncture, herbal remedies, and mind-body practices, offer additional options for treating diabetes and boosting general well-being.

One strategy to merge standard and complementary therapies in diabetes control is through a personalized treatment plan suited to the individual's needs and preferences. Healthcare providers can work cooperatively with persons with diabetes to establish a complete strategy that blends conventional treatments with complementary therapies based on their unique health objectives, preferences, and cultural beliefs. This technique provides a more holistic and tailored approach to care that covers the physical, emotional, and psychological elements of diabetes control.

Incorporating complementary therapies into diabetes care can potentially bring extra benefits beyond blood sugar control. For example, acupuncture has been demonstrated to increase insulin sensitivity and minimize diabetes-related problems such as neuropathy and retinopathy. Herbal medicines, such as cinnamon and fenugreek, may have potential benefits for blood sugar management and insulin sensitivity when used as supplementary therapies. Mind-body methods, such as yoga and mindfulness meditation, can help reduce stress, increase sleep quality, and promote general well-being, which are significant aspects of treating diabetes.

Furthermore, integrating traditional and complementary medicines in diabetes management involves collaboration and communication among healthcare providers, including physicians, nurses, dietitians, and alternative healthcare practitioners. By working together as a team, healthcare providers may guarantee that patients with diabetes receive comprehensive and coordinated treatment that accommodates their diverse needs and preferences. This interdisciplinary approach enables for the sharing of knowledge and skills across multiple healthcare specialties, leading to improved health outcomes for patients with diabetes.

It's crucial to note that while complementary therapies can offer additional alternatives for managing diabetes, they should be used in conjunction with, not as a replacement for, standard medical treatments. Individuals with diabetes should always contact their healthcare professional before adopting complementary therapies into their treatment plan to ensure safety and effectiveness, especially if they are taking medicines or insulin.

Integrating traditional and complementary therapies in diabetes care gives a holistic approach that recognizes the various requirements of individuals and complements standard medical treatments. By incorporating complementary therapies into personalized treatment plans, healthcare providers can provide comprehensive and individualized care that addresses the physical, emotional, and psychological aspects of diabetes management, ultimately improving health outcomes and value of life for individuals with diabetes.

Patient-Centered Care and Shared Decision-Making

Patient-centered care and shared decision-making are fundamental ideas in modern healthcare that prioritize the needs, interests, and values of patients in the decision-making process about their health and treatment alternatives. This approach recognizes that patients are unique persons with their objectives, beliefs, and values and that they should be actively involved in choices concerning their care.

At the basis of patient-centered care is the idea of treating patients as partners in their healthcare journey. This requires engaging patients in open and honest conversation, listening to their concerns, and supporting their autonomy and right to make educated choices about their health. Healthcare providers who practice patient-centered care try to develop trusted and collaborative relationships with their patients, where mutual respect and understanding are key.

Shared decision-making is a crucial component of patient-centered care and comprises a collaborative process between healthcare providers and patients to reach decisions about treatment alternatives that match the patient's values and preferences. In shared decision-making, healthcare providers give patients with information about their diagnosis, prognosis, and available treatment options, including the potential benefits, dangers, and alternatives. Patients are then enabled to weigh the facts and actively engage in the decision-making process by expressing their preferences, concerns, and aspirations.

By integrating patients in the decision-making process, shared decision-making develops a sense of ownership and empowerment, which can lead to higher satisfaction with care and better adherence to treatment programs. It also promotes a more individualized approach to care that takes into consideration the particular requirements and circumstances of each patient. Shared decision-making is particularly crucial in the management of chronic illnesses like diabetes, where treatment plans may require complex pharmaceutical regimens, lifestyle modifications, and continuing self-management.

Patient-centered care and shared decision-making are essential principles in modern healthcare that prioritize the needs, interests, and values of patients in the decision-making process about their health and treatment alternatives. By fostering open communication, mutual respect, and collaboration between healthcare practitioners and patients, these principles support a more individualized and empowering approach to care that ultimately leads to improved health outcomes and patient satisfaction.

Role of Technology in Integrative Diabetes Management

The role of technology in integrated diabetes treatment is constantly evolving, enabling innovative ways to enhance the care and support accessible to those living with diabetes. From wearable gadgets to mobile applications and telemedicine platforms, technology has the potential to change how diabetes is monitored, managed, and treated.

One of the important contributions of technology to integrated diabetes management is in the area of continuous glucose monitoring (CGM). CGM systems use sensors to detect blood sugar levels in real-time, providing individuals with useful insights into their glucose changes throughout the day. This real-time data enables more proactive management of diabetes, enabling individuals to make timely adjustments to their diet, medication, and lifestyle choices to maintain optimal blood sugar control.

Another key feature of technology in integrative diabetes treatment is the use of mobile applications and digital platforms to track and manage many aspects of diabetes care. These programs can help individuals check their blood sugar levels, track their food intake and physical activity, set reminders for medication dosages, and even connect with healthcare specialists for virtual consultations and support. By offering simple access to individualized information and resources, these digital solutions empower individuals to take a more active part in managing their diabetes and making educated decisions about their health.

Telemedicine has also emerged as a helpful tool in integrated diabetes management, especially in the context of remote or underprivileged populations where access to standard healthcare services may be limited. Telemedicine systems enable users to consult with healthcare providers, including endocrinologists, diabetes educators, and nutritionists, through virtual visits and telehealth consultations. This online access to care helps transcend geographical barriers and guarantees that persons with diabetes receive prompt and individualized support regardless of their location.

In addition to monitoring and management tools, technology has also permitted the development of revolutionary treatment alternatives for diabetes. For example, insulin pumps and automated insulin delivery systems use advanced algorithms and sensor technologies to give exact dosages of insulin based on real-time glucose readings, simulating the function of a healthy pancreas. These devices allow persons with diabetes better flexibility and control over their insulin delivery, leading to improved blood sugar management and quality of life.

Overall, technology plays a vital role in integrated diabetes management by enabling patients with diabetes access to enhanced monitoring equipment, digital platforms for self-management, telemedicine services, and innovative treatment alternatives. By embracing the power of technology, healthcare providers and patients alike may work together to enhance diabetes care and improve health outcomes in the rapidly developing healthcare landscape.

Chapter 5

Addressing Diabetes Complications and Comorbidities

The care of diabetes complications and comorbidities is an essential component of comprehensive diabetes management. This is due to the fact that people who have diabetes are at a greater risk of developing a variety of health problems that go beyond elevated blood sugar levels. It is necessary to have a comprehensive understanding of these complications and to take preventative measures to manage them to ensure that diabetes care is holistic.

The control of cardiovascular risk factors is one of the key focuses in the process of resolving issues associated with diabetes. People who have diabetes are at a greater risk of developing cardiovascular complications such as heart disease, stroke, and other cardiovascular issues. As a result, the management of blood pressure and cholesterol levels, as well as the adoption of lifestyle choices that are beneficial to the heart, such as engaging in regular physical activity and maintaining a balanced diet, are fundamental components in the reduction of cardiovascular risks associated with diabetes.

Another important factor to take into account is the effect that diabetes has on the health of the kidneys. The condition known as diabetic nephropathy, which is a kind of kidney disease, is a common consequence that requires careful monitoring of kidney function with diagnostic testing and checkups at regular intervals. The management of blood pressure, the control of blood sugar levels, and the adoption of a diet that is kidney-friendly are all essential components in the process of maintaining kidney health in diabetics.

The need to have routine eye exams is highlighted by the fact that diabetic retinopathy and other diseases associated with diabetes can affect the eyes. The prevention or reduction of visual loss can be achieved through early detection and intervention. Maintaining stable blood sugar levels, regulating blood pressure, and refraining from smoking are critical steps to safeguard eye health in adults with diabetes.

Nerve damage, or diabetic neuropathy, is another problem that can affect numerous sections of the body. Foot care becomes particularly critical, as patients with diabetes may feel diminished sensation or circulation in their feet, increasing the risk of infections and ulcers. Regular foot inspections, suitable footwear, and rigorous foot cleaning are vital in preventing issues connected to diabetic neuropathy.

Furthermore, addressing mental health elements is vital in the setting of diabetic problems. The everyday management issues and the chronic nature of the ailment can add to stress, anxiety, and depression. Incorporating mental health assistance into diabetes care, such as counseling or support groups, can dramatically enhance overall well-being and improve the individual's capacity to cope with the challenges of living with diabetes.

Comorbidities, or the coexistence of other health disorders with diabetes, further underscore the necessity for a holistic healthcare approach. Conditions like obesity, hypertension, and sleep apnea often co-occur with diabetes and require coordinated management measures. Lifestyle adjustments, medication management, and regular health screenings are key components in addressing chronic comorbidities and achieving optimal health outcomes.

Addressing diabetes complications and comorbidities entails a multi-faceted approach that spans cardiovascular health, kidney function, eye care, nerve health, mental well-being, and the management of coexisting health disorders. Through proactive monitoring, lifestyle adjustments, and tailored healthcare plans, individuals with diabetes can limit the burden of complications and comorbidities, leading to improved overall health and quality of life.

Macrovascular Complications

Macrovascular complications of diabetes relate to major health disorders that affect large blood vessels throughout the body, including the heart and the blood vessels that give oxygen and nutrition to the limbs. These problems can have major repercussions and require cautious management to limit their influence on general health.

One of the most well-known macrovascular consequences of diabetes is cardiovascular disease. Diabetes dramatically raises the chance of developing heart disease, including illnesses such as coronary artery disease, heart attack, and stroke. High blood sugar levels over time can damage blood vessels and contribute to the accumulation of plaque, a fatty substance that narrows and hardens the arteries, leading to restricted blood flow to the heart and brain. As a result, patients with diabetes are more prone to experiencing cardiovascular events and require attentive monitoring and control of risk factors such as high blood pressure, high cholesterol, and smoking.

Peripheral vascular disease is another macrovascular consequence of diabetes that affects the blood vessels outside of the heart and brain, particularly those delivering blood to the legs and feet. Individuals with diabetes are at a higher risk of developing peripheral vascular disease due to the same factors that contribute to cardiovascular disease, namely, damage to blood vessels induced by high blood sugar levels. Peripheral vascular disease can lead to impaired circulation, numbness, discomfort, and slow-healing wounds in the lower extremities. In severe situations, it can result in critical limb ischemia, a condition where blood flow to the limbs is severely reduced, increasing the risk of amputation.

Effective care of macrovascular complications of diabetes entails a comprehensive approach that tackles underlying risk factors and supports overall cardiovascular health. This may involve lifestyle alterations such as adopting a heart-healthy diet, engaging in regular physical activity, keeping a healthy weight, and stopping smoking. Additionally, drugs to lower blood pressure and cholesterol levels, as well as blood-thinning medications to reduce the risk of blood clots, may be administered to manage cardiovascular and peripheral vascular disease.

Regular medical check-ups and screenings are critical for the early detection and management of macrovascular problems in patients with diabetes. Monitoring blood sugar levels, blood pressure, cholesterol levels, and renal function, as well as doing frequent foot inspections, can assist in identifying potential difficulties early and avoiding the advancement of disorders. By taking proactive actions to address macrovascular problems and manage underlying risk factors, individuals with diabetes can lower their risk of major cardiovascular events and maintain their overall health and well-being.

Microvascular Complications

Microvascular complications of diabetes relate to issues that affect the small blood vessels throughout the body. These problems can have catastrophic effects and require cautious management to prevent long-term difficulties. Three common microvascular consequences of diabetes include diabetic retinopathy, diabetic neuropathy, and diabetic nephropathy.

Diabetic retinopathy is a consequence of diabetes that affects the eyes and is a primary cause of blindness in adults. It occurs when high blood sugar levels damage the blood vessels in the retina, the light-sensitive tissue in the back of the eye. As a result, the blood vessels may leak fluid or bleed, leading to blurred vision, floaters, and finally vision loss if left untreated. Regular eye exams and early management are critical for treating diabetic retinopathy and preventing vision loss.

Diabetic neuropathy is a type of nerve injury that can arise as a result of diabetes. It most usually affects the nerves in the feet and legs, although it can also affect other regions of the body. Diabetic neuropathy can cause symptoms such as numbness, tingling, pain, and weakness in the affected areas. In severe situations, it can lead to consequences such as foot ulcers and amputations. Managing blood sugar levels, maintaining a healthy lifestyle, and taking drugs to treat symptoms are critical measures for preventing and managing diabetic neuropathy.

Diabetic nephropathy is a consequence of diabetes that affects the kidneys and is a significant cause of kidney failure. It occurs when high blood sugar levels damage the blood vessels in the kidneys, leading to diminished kidney function over time. Diabetic nephropathy may initially show no symptoms, but as it progresses, it can cause symptoms such as edema in the legs, increased urination, and weariness. Controlling blood sugar levels, regulating blood pressure, and maintaining a healthy lifestyle are critical for preventing and managing diabetic nephropathy.

Overall, microvascular consequences of diabetes, including diabetic retinopathy, neuropathy, and nephropathy, can have substantial repercussions for an individual's health and quality of life. Early detection and management are crucial to preventing long-term problems and sustaining overall health. Regular medical check-ups, eye exams, foot care, and adherence to prescribed treatment plans are critical components of treating microvascular problems in patients with diabetes.

Psychosocial Complications and Mental Health Considerations

Psychosocial problems and mental health considerations are essential parts of diabetes management that typically receive less attention but are equally important for overall well-being. Living with diabetes can bring different issues that transcend physical health, impacting an individual's emotional and psychological state.

One of the key psychosocial consequences linked to diabetes is the emotional toll of treating a chronic condition. The everyday chores of monitoring blood sugar levels, sticking to medication regimens, and making lifestyle adjustments can be burdensome and frustrating. Individuals with diabetes may experience feelings of frustration, worry, or sadness as they navigate the complexity of their condition. Moreover, the worry of consequences and the frequent need to make health-related decisions can take a toll on one's mental health.

Stigma and misconceptions around diabetes can also contribute to psychosocial consequences. Society's perception of diabetes as a result of bad lifestyle choices or lack of self-control can contribute to feelings of shame or guilt among those with the condition. Additionally, the fear of being judged or discriminated against owing to their diabetes condition may lead to social isolation and a reluctance to seek support.

Furthermore, diabetes management can affect several elements of an individual's life, including relationships, jobs, and leisure activities. Balancing diabetes care with other responsibilities and commitments can be tough, leading to stress and pressure in interpersonal relationships. Additionally, controlling diabetes in the workplace or social settings may need concessions and adaptations that might impair an individual's sense of inclusion and belonging.

Addressing psychosocial problems and mental health considerations in diabetes care demands a holistic approach that blends physical, emotional, and psychological well-being. Healthcare practitioners play a critical role in supporting patients with diabetes by addressing their psychological needs and providing access to appropriate resources and support services.

Incorporating techniques to boost mental health and well-being is vital in diabetes management. This may involve counseling or therapy to address emotional issues, support groups to connect with people facing similar circumstances, and stress-management approaches such as mindfulness or relaxation exercises. Additionally, establishing open communication and offering knowledge about diabetes to dispel stereotypes and eliminate stigma can help individuals feel more empowered and supported in managing their illness.

Recognizing and resolving psychosocial problems and mental health considerations are key parts of comprehensive diabetes management. By addressing the emotional and psychological impact of diabetes and offering appropriate support and resources, individuals with diabetes can better cope with the challenges of their condition and enhance their overall quality of life.

Multimorbidity Management in Diabetes Care

Managing multiple conditions, commonly known as multimorbidity, alongside diabetes demands a thorough and coordinated approach to care. Multimorbidity refers to the existence of two or more chronic illnesses in an individual, which might complicate diabetes management and increase the complexity of treatment strategies. Effectively treating multimorbidity in diabetes treatment includes addressing the particular demands and problems associated with each condition while providing coordinated and patient-centered care.

One of the main concerns in multimorbidity management is the prioritization of treatment goals depending on individual patient preferences and overall health conditions. Healthcare providers engage cooperatively with patients to set realistic treatment goals that take into consideration their choices, values, and priorities. This patient-centered approach helps guarantee that treatment programs are adjusted to match the specific needs and preferences of each individual, including criteria such as age, comorbidities, and lifestyle factors.

Another significant feature of multimorbidity management in diabetes care is the integration of care across multiple healthcare providers and locations. Coordinated care entails good communication and coordination among primary care physicians, specialists, nurses, pharmacists, and other healthcare providers involved in the care of patients with diabetes and multiple comorbidities. This interdisciplinary approach helps guarantee that patients receive comprehensive and integrated care that covers all of their health requirements.

Additionally, addressing multimorbidity in diabetes care involves an emphasis on preventive care and health promotion. This includes regular monitoring of critical health indicators, such as blood pressure, cholesterol levels, and renal function, to detect and address possible issues early. Healthcare practitioners often emphasize the need for lifestyle adjustments, such as adopting a nutritious diet, engaging in regular physical activity, and quitting smoking, to lower the risk of problems and improve overall health outcomes.

Furthermore, medication management is an important component of multimorbidity treatment in diabetes therapy. Healthcare providers carefully assess the potential interactions between drugs used to treat diabetes and other comorbidities to minimize the risk of side effects and enhance treatment outcomes. Patient education and medication adherence assistance are also crucial to ensuring that patients understand their treatment regimens and can stick to them properly.

Managing multimorbidity in diabetes care demands a holistic and patient-centered approach that incorporates the specific requirements and preferences of each individual. By prioritizing treatment goals, integrating care across healthcare providers and settings, emphasizing preventive care and health promotion, and optimizing medication management, healthcare providers can effectively manage multiple health conditions in patients with diabetes and improve overall health outcomes.

Chapter 6

Prevention Strategies and Public Health Initiatives

Prevention strategies and public health programs play a significant role in combating the growing burden of diabetes and decreasing its impact on individuals and communities. These projects attempt to encourage healthy behaviors, raise awareness of diabetes risk factors, and create supportive environments that facilitate good lifestyle choices.

One of the important prevention techniques is promoting healthy eating behaviors and encouraging the consumption of a balanced diet rich in fruits, vegetables, whole grains, and lean proteins while reducing the consumption of processed foods, sugary beverages, and harmful fats. Public health campaigns and educational programs can help individuals make informed food choices and adopt better eating patterns, which can reduce the chance of developing type 2 diabetes and improve overall health outcomes.

Another key part of prevention is promoting regular physical activity and encouraging individuals to engage in regular exercise. Physical activity not only helps maintain a healthy weight but also increases insulin sensitivity and lowers the risk of acquiring type 2 diabetes. Public health initiatives can include initiatives such as community-based exercise programs, workplace wellness initiatives, and school-based physical education programs to encourage individuals of all ages to be physically active and include regular exercise in their daily routines.

In addition to promoting good food and physical activity, public health campaigns also focus on raising knowledge of diabetes risk factors and encouraging early identification through regular testing. Educational campaigns can include information about the necessity of keeping a healthy weight, managing blood sugar levels, and monitoring blood pressure and cholesterol levels. By improving awareness about the risk factors for diabetes and the necessity of early detection, these campaigns can help individuals take proactive steps to prevent or manage the condition effectively.

Furthermore, public health programs strive to establish supportive environments that make it easier for individuals to make healthy lifestyle choices. This may include rules and regulations that promote access to healthy meals, stimulate the construction of safe and accessible recreational venues for physical activity, and support workplace wellness initiatives. By building conditions that support healthy behaviors, public health programs can help lower the burden of diabetes and improve population health outcomes.

Prevention methods and public health programs are crucial components of efforts to combat the diabetes epidemic and improve health and well-being. By promoting good eating habits, encouraging regular physical activity, raising awareness about diabetes risk factors, and establishing supportive environments, these efforts can help individuals and communities prevent or manage diabetes effectively and improve overall health outcomes.

Primary Prevention of Type 2 Diabetes

Primary prevention of type 2 diabetes is critical for reducing the incidence of the disease and improving population health outcomes. This involves implementing measures aimed at avoiding the onset of diabetes in those who are at high risk due to lifestyle factors or other predisposing factors.

Lifestyle Interventions:

At the core of type 2 diabetes prevention lies the potential for lifestyle adjustments. These therapies emphasize developing and sustaining a healthy lifestyle through changes in eating habits, physical exercise, and overall behavior. For instance, advocating a diet rich in natural foods, vegetables, and lean proteins, while avoiding the intake of processed sweets and harmful fats is crucial. Regular physical activity also takes primacy, not just as a technique for weight control but as an effective instrument for boosting insulin sensitivity.

Crucially, lifestyle changes reach beyond individual choices. Public health programs play a crucial role, in increasing community-wide awareness and facilitating supportive conditions. Communities that prioritize access to nutritional meals, stimulate physical activity through well-designed urban areas, and promote workplace wellness contribute greatly to the success of primary preventive programs.

Pharmaceutical Approaches: In certain circumstances, especially for persons with a higher risk of developing type 2 diabetes, pharmaceutical therapies provide a beneficial addition to lifestyle adjustments. Medications aiming to reduce blood glucose levels, boost insulin sensitivity, or address underlying metabolic abnormalities may be advised. However, it's vital to highlight that these medicinal interventions are not standalone remedies but work best in unison with lifestyle improvements.

Pharmacological therapies require careful assessment, taking into account an individual's overall health, existing medical disorders, and potential adverse effects. Healthcare professionals play a significant role in personalizing pharmaceutical therapies for each patient, ensuring a personalized and effective strategy.

While these approaches—lifestyle interventions and pharmaceutical strategies—stand as separate pillars in the primary prevention of type 2 diabetes, their true strength appears when merged. A holistic strategy, combining the power of informed lifestyle choices with tailored pharmacological support, holds the potential for a more effective and lasting solution to the rising challenge of type 2 diabetes.

The prevention of type 2 diabetes includes developing comprehensive measures that target both lifestyle factors and other risk factors involved with the development of the illness. By promoting healthy behaviors and offering tailored interventions to people at high risk, primary preventive programs can help lower the incidence of type 2 diabetes and improve overall health outcomes in population

Screening and Early Detection Programs

Screening and early detection programs are an important part of public health initiatives aimed at identifying individuals at risk of acquiring various health disorders, including diabetes. These programs are meant to identify persons with prediabetes or early stages of diabetes who may benefit from early intervention to prevent or delay the onset of the illness and its complications.

One of the key objectives of screening and early detection programs is to identify individuals who may have undiagnosed diabetes or prediabetes, as early diagnosis allows for early intervention and management. These programs frequently utilize proven screening technologies, including fasting blood glucose testing, oral glucose tolerance tests, and HbA1c tests, to identify patients at risk. Additionally, risk assessment questionnaires and electronic health records may be utilized to identify individuals who may benefit from further testing.

Early identification of diabetes is crucial because it allows for the prompt adoption of therapies targeted at reducing or delaying the evolution of the illness and its consequences. Lifestyle therapies, such as dietary adjustments, increased physical activity, and weight control, are typically indicated for patients with prediabetes to help prevent or delay the onset of type 2 diabetes. For persons with diabetes, early detection allows for the immediate beginning of appropriate medical therapy and continued care to prevent complications and enhance health outcomes.

Screening and early detection programs are frequently conducted at several levels of the healthcare system, including primary care settings, community health centers, and public health programs. These programs may target certain populations at increased risk of acquiring diabetes, such as persons with a family history of diabetes, individuals who are overweight or obese, or those with certain ethnic or racial origins known to be at higher risk.

In addition to detecting persons with undiagnosed diabetes or prediabetes, screening, and early detection programs also play a significant role in promoting awareness about diabetes risk factors and encouraging individuals to seek appropriate medical care and lifestyle modifications. By identifying persons at risk and promoting early intervention, these programs assist in decreasing the burden of diabetes and improving health outcomes on a community level.

The interaction of diabetes management and health policy is a dynamic force that impacts the accessibility, affordability, and quality of care for persons coping with this condition. Advocacy initiatives aiming at influencing health policies play a crucial role in managing the problems and opportunities within this sector.

Health policies, comparable to the compass directing a ship through uncharted waters, establish the route for the delivery of diabetes care on a broader social scale. Advocacy activities strive to not only steer this compass but also to modify its calibration, ensuring that policies align with the increasing needs of persons afflicted by diabetes. It's a complex tango between the subtleties of healthcare delivery and the regulatory structures that govern it.

Advocates advocate the cause of equitable access to diabetes care, relentlessly striving to break down barriers that may obstruct persons from accessing timely and effective treatment. They work with legislators to promote the necessity of preventive measures, early detection programs, and comprehensive management solutions. The aim is not only to lobby for change but to construct a healthcare landscape where individuals with diabetes find supportive and accessible services.

In this advocacy journey, storytellers emerge as powerful narrators, weaving narratives that humanize the impact of diabetes on individuals, families, and communities. These stories become catalysts for change, providing a vivid picture that resonates with policymakers and the larger public. They translate numbers into relatable experiences, boosting empathy and understanding.

Furthermore, lobbying efforts extend beyond the policy area, entering into the center of public conversation. Social media platforms become battlegrounds where campaigners raise their voices, shedding awareness on diabetes-related difficulties and rallying support. It's a digital agora where conversations transcend the clinical, delving into the lived experiences of those navigating the maze of diabetes treatment.

The synergy between health policy and advocacy is not a one-size-fits-all answer but rather an evolving narrative where collective voices define the outlines of diabetes care. It's about disrupting the existing quo, encouraging politicians to envisage a healthcare environment that prioritizes prevention, embraces innovation, and serves the holistic needs of persons living with diabetes.

In the unfolding chapters of healthcare advocacy, the goal is not simply to influence legislation but to build a narrative where diabetes care is not a distant shore but an accessible vista. Through concerted efforts, advocates try to establish a healthcare environment that recognizes the particular problems posed by diabetes and, in doing so, contributes to the well-being of individuals and the community at large.

Community-Based Interventions for Diabetes Prevention

In the bustling neighborhoods and lively communities that comprise our society, community-based interventions emerge as beacons of hope in the fight against diabetes. These treatments, like seeds placed in fertile soil, take root and blossom into transformative initiatives that nourish healthier lifestyles and develop supportive environments for those at risk of diabetes.

Picture this: a bustling community center where persons from all walks of life come to begin a shared journey toward well-being. Here, health educators and community leaders arrange a symphony of activities, from participatory workshops on healthy cuisine to group fitness classes that fire the spirit of friendship. It's a rich tapestry of colors and cultures, where the united objective of diabetes prevention joins disparate voices in harmony.

Community gardens, analogous to verdant oases within metropolitan environments, offer more than just a cornucopia of fresh produce. They serve as living classrooms where folks learn about the connection between nutrition and health, developing not just fruits and vegetables but also a deeper understanding of how dietary choices affect well-being. As hands dig into the soil and hearts connect over shared experiences, friendships are built that transcend the limits of age, ethnicity, and socioeconomic class.

Beyond the physical world, community-based treatments dive into the realm of social support and empowerment. Support groups, comparable to lighthouses guiding ships through stormy seas, provide a safe harbor for persons coping with the emotional toll of diabetes. Here, memories are shared, tears are shed, and laughter resonates through the room as folks find peace in knowing they are not alone on their path.

Innovative techniques, such as mobile health clinics and community health fairs, deliver healthcare right to the doorstep of underserved areas. These mobile units, equipped with state-of-the-art technology and staffed by compassionate healthcare professionals, bridge the gap between healthcare services and those who need them most. It's healthcare on wheels, breaking down barriers of access and allowing individuals to take responsibility for their health.

Schools, churches, and businesses become epicenters of health promotion, where wellness activities penetrate the fabric of daily life. From nutrition education programs in schools to corporate wellness challenges that promote friendly rivalry, these settings become catalysts for change, establishing a culture of health that goes far beyond the bounds of typical healthcare settings.

As the sun sets on another day in the community, the influence of these initiatives reverberates through the streets and alleyways. Individuals empowered with information, encouraged by their peers, and equipped with the means for healthier living take timid steps towards a brighter, healthier future. And with this community-driven approach to diabetes prevention, the seeds of change take root, flowering into a landscape where health and well-being flourish.

Chapter 7

Innovations in Diabetes Research and Technology

In the world of diabetes research and technology, ongoing innovation pulls us ahead on a road of discovery and advancement. These innovations, like beacons of progress, illumine the path towards more effective control and treatment of diabetes.

Imagine a world where glucose monitoring is not simply a task, but a seamless part of everyday life. Continuous glucose monitoring (CGM) devices, equipped with cutting-edge sensors and wireless connectivity, provide real-time data on blood sugar levels, helping persons with diabetes to make informed decisions about their health. No more finger pricks or guessing - just reliable insights at your fingertips.

The emergence of artificial pancreas devices heralds a new era in diabetes management, as technology smoothly mimics the function of the pancreas to regulate blood sugar levels. These closed-loop devices, comprising an insulin pump and continuous glucose monitor, work in harmony to provide exact dosages of insulin based on real-time data, freeing users from the stress of constant attention and manual changes.

In the field of medication, innovative pharmacotherapies offer intriguing prospects for more targeted and individualized therapeutic methods. From breakthrough oral antidiabetic drugs that promote insulin sensitivity to injectable therapies that imitate the effect of incretin hormones, these advancements provide new tools in the arsenal against diabetes, bringing promise for improved glycemic control and lower risk of complications.

Beyond standard treatment modalities, innovative technologies are altering the landscape of diabetes care. From mobile health applications that track nutrition and exercise to wearable devices that monitor vital signs and activity levels, the incorporation of technology into diabetes management is altering the way we handle this chronic condition. These tools not only enable persons with diabetes to take charge of their health but also facilitate more individualized and proactive care.

In the area of science, innovative investigations uncover new insights into the underlying mechanisms of diabetes and prospective targets for treatments. From dissecting the genetic foundation of monogenic diabetes to uncovering the complicated interplay between environmental factors and disease risk, these discoveries pave the path for more focused and effective prevention efforts.

Innovations in diabetes science and technology provide the possibility of a brighter future for persons living with this chronic condition. As scientists, engineers, and healthcare professionals unite to push the boundaries of knowledge and technology, we get ever closer to a world where diabetes is not just treated but defeated.

Advances in Diabetes Genetics and Precision Medicine

In recent years, substantial advancements have been achieved in understanding the genetic foundations of diabetes, paving the door for the advent of precision medicine treatments tailored to individual individuals. Genetic research has revealed multiple genetic variations related to diabetes susceptibility, providing vital insights into the complicated genetic architecture of the illness.

One of the most important achievements in diabetes genetics is the identification of particular genes implicated in both type 1 and type 2 diabetes. Genome-wide association studies (GWAS) have discovered hundreds of genetic loci related to diabetes risk, offering information on the underlying biochemical mechanisms involved in disease development.

Furthermore, developments in sequencing technology, such as next-generation sequencing (NGS), have enabled researchers to investigate the full genetic landscape of diabetes in unprecedented detail. Whole-genome sequencing and whole-exome sequencing have permitted the detection of uncommon genetic variations with potentially substantial consequences for diabetes risk and management.

In addition to genetic research, precision medicine approaches aim to utilize individual genetic information to adapt treatment strategies for optimal outcomes. Pharmacogenomics, for instance, focuses on how genetic variants influence an individual's reaction to drugs used in diabetes control. By finding genetic markers that predict treatment responses or unfavorable drug reactions, healthcare providers can personalize pharmaceutical regimens to maximize efficacy and decrease side effects.

Moreover, genetic testing and risk stratification techniques enable healthcare providers to identify patients at elevated risk of acquiring diabetes or its complications. This proactive strategy allows for early intervention and focused preventative interventions, such as lifestyle modifications and individualized screening regimens, to minimize disease progression and enhance long-term health outcomes.

The integration of genetics and precision medicine into diabetes care holds considerable promise for increasing our understanding of the illness and optimizing treatment methods. By uncovering the genetic complexity of diabetes and adapting therapies to individual genetic profiles, we can move closer to creating tailored and successful management solutions for people with diabetes.

Novel Therapeutic Targets and Drug Development

Ongoing research continues to find novel therapeutic targets and accelerate drug development, bringing new hope for improved treatment alternatives. These efforts are driven by a detailed understanding of the underlying molecular mechanisms of diabetes and the discovery of critical pathways implicated in disease etiology.

One potential field of study is addressing inflammation and immunological dysregulation, which are known to contribute to the development and progression of diabetes. By modifying inflammatory pathways and immunological responses, researchers attempt to ameliorate beta-cell failure and insulin resistance, thus potentially preventing or reducing disease development.

Furthermore, the gut microbiota has emerged as a potential therapeutic target in diabetes control. Studies have revealed that variations in gut bacteria composition and function might influence metabolic health and contribute to the development of insulin resistance and obesity. Novel therapies targeted at altering the gut microbiota, such as probiotics, prebiotics, and fecal microbiota transplantation, have promise for improving glucose metabolism and insulin sensitivity.

In addition to addressing specific routes and mechanisms, researchers are researching new drug delivery technologies to enhance the efficacy and safety of diabetic therapy. Nanotechnology-based drug delivery systems, for example, offer the promise of targeted and controlled release of insulin and other therapeutic medicines, minimizing adverse effects and boosting patient adherence.

Moreover, the advent of precision medicine has paved the path for personalized therapy approaches suited to specific patients' genetic profiles and metabolic features. By identifying genetic variations and biomarkers related to diabetes risk and treatment response, healthcare providers can optimize drug selection and dose, leading to more effective and individualized diabetes management.

In conclusion, ongoing research into novel therapeutic targets and medication development holds significant promise for enhancing diabetes care. By targeting specific pathways, utilizing the potential of the gut microbiome, exploring innovative drug delivery technologies, and adopting precision medicine, researchers are seeking to enhance treatment options and outcomes for persons living with diabetes.

Digital Health Solutions for Diabetes Management

The integration of digital health technologies has altered the way individuals monitor, track, and control their condition. These technological developments give a real-time and tailored approach to diabetes management, empowering patients and healthcare practitioners alike.

One major digital breakthrough is the emergence of continuous glucose monitoring (CGM) systems. These devices offer people with diabetes a comprehensive view of their glucose levels throughout the day, enabling them to make informed decisions regarding their nutrition, physical activity, and insulin delivery. The real-time data given by CGM devices not only aids glycemic management but also leads to a better understanding of how various circumstances influence blood sugar levels.

Mobile applications customized for diabetes management have become important tools for users trying to optimize their everyday activities. These apps generally integrate features such as meal tracking, medication reminders, and activity monitoring, supporting a holistic approach to diabetes self-care. Users can quickly submit their data, obtain insights, and exchange information with healthcare practitioners, fostering collaborative and patient-centered treatment.

Telemedicine has emerged as a game-changer in diabetes management, notably in enhancing accessibility to healthcare services. Virtual consultations enable individuals to visit with diabetes specialists from the comfort of their homes, promoting timely interventions and decreasing barriers to regular medical check-ups. The convenience of telemedicine is particularly advantageous for persons in remote or underserved locations.

Wearable gadgets, like smart insulin pens and insulin pumps, contribute to the seamless integration of technology into diabetes management. These devices not only ease insulin administration but also provide extra data points for better therapy modifications. The user-friendly interfaces of these devices increase the entire diabetes experience, making it more intuitive and less obtrusive.

Artificial intelligence (AI) algorithms play a vital role in interpreting the massive statistics created by digital health solutions. These algorithms can forecast glucose trends, recognize patterns, and offer individualized recommendations for better diabetes management. Machine learning applications continue to advance, promising more accurate and tailored insights for users.

The digital transformation in diabetes care is bringing forth a new era of empowerment and efficiency. From continuous glucose monitoring to mobile applications, telemedicine, wearables, and AI-driven solutions, the integration of digital health is building a future where managing diabetes is not only successful but also suited to each individual's specific requirements and preferences.

Wearable Devices and Remote Monitoring Technologies

Wearable devices and remote monitoring technologies have evolved as crucial components of modern healthcare, particularly in the field of chronic disease management. These revolutionary solutions allow individuals the capacity to measure several health variables in real-time, providing vital insights into their well-being and enabling proactive interventions.

One of the most popular instances of wearable technology in healthcare is the smartwatch. Equipped with sensors to measure heart rate, activity levels, and even blood oxygen saturation, smartwatches serve as convenient and unobtrusive tools for continuous health monitoring. Users may conveniently track their physical activity, sleep habits, and vital signs, allowing them a thorough assessment of their overall health state.

Beyond smartwatches, wearable fitness trackers have gained popularity for their capacity to encourage and monitor physical activity. These gadgets provide users with real-time feedback on their exercise regimens, step counts, and calorie expenditure, inspiring consumers to adopt better lifestyles. By stimulating regular physical exercise, wearable fitness trackers contribute to the prevention and management of chronic illnesses such as obesity and cardiovascular disease.

Remote monitoring technologies enable healthcare providers to monitor patients' health state from a distance, facilitating prompt treatments and reducing the need for frequent in-person visits. For those with chronic diseases like diabetes or hypertension, remote monitoring devices allow for continuous observation of crucial health indicators such as blood glucose levels or blood pressure. By communicating data to healthcare practitioners in real-time, these technologies enable proactive alterations to treatment programs, ultimately improving patient outcomes and decreasing the burden of illness management.

Implantable devices represent another frontier in wearable technology, allowing continuous monitoring and treatments for those with chronic diseases. For example, implantable cardiac monitors can detect and record aberrant heart rhythms, providing critical diagnostic information for individuals with arrhythmias or other cardiac diseases. Similarly, implantable insulin pumps allow accurate insulin delivery for persons with diabetes, replicating the function of a healthy pancreas and improving glycemic control.

Wearable gadgets and remote monitoring technologies are transforming healthcare by empowering individuals to take control of their health and enabling healthcare practitioners to give more personalized and proactive care. From smartwatches and fitness trackers to remote monitoring devices and implantable technology, these breakthroughs are transforming the way we monitor, manage, and treat chronic conditions.

Chapter 8

Future Directions and Challenges in Diabetes Care

As we look to the future of diabetes care, there are various potential directions and difficulties that lie ahead. One prominent area of attention is the continuous growth of customized medicine and precision therapy. With developments in genetics, biomarkers, and data analytics, healthcare providers may adapt treatment approaches to individual patients, optimizing outcomes and lowering the risk of consequences.

Furthermore, the inclusion of digital health technologies holds enormous potential in improving diabetes care. From wearable gadgets and smartphone apps to telehealth platforms and artificial intelligence, these solutions offer remote monitoring, real-time data analysis, and personalized therapies. By harnessing these technologies, healthcare providers can increase patient involvement, better illness management, and promote quicker interventions.

Another key component of future diabetes care is the emphasis on preventative methods and public health management. By addressing socioeconomic determinants of health, supporting healthy lifestyle practices, and adopting community-based interventions, healthcare systems can lower the incidence of diabetes and its related problems. Moreover, proactive screening and early detection programs can identify persons at high risk of developing diabetes, allowing for prompt interventions and risk mitigation.

However, despite these breakthroughs and potential, significant obstacles continue in the field of diabetes care. One important concern is the increased prevalence of diabetes worldwide, driven by factors such as aging populations, urbanization, and sedentary lifestyles. This presents a huge burden on healthcare systems, necessitating creative methods to disease management and resource allocation.

Additionally, inequities in access to healthcare and diabetes management remain a major concern, particularly in marginalized neighborhoods and low-income populations. Addressing these inequities requires a holistic approach that incorporates healthcare policy reform, community participation, and tailored interventions to increase access to quality care and support services.

likewise, the expanding environment of healthcare legislation, reimbursement schemes, and technology developments offers problems for healthcare practitioners and policymakers alike. Striking a balance between stimulating innovation, ensuring patient safety, and maintaining cost and accessibility of diabetes care is vital for sustainable growth in the field.

The future of diabetes care has enormous promise with developments in tailored medicine, digital health technologies, and preventive initiatives. However, tackling obstacles such as increased prevalence, healthcare inequities, and regulatory complications will require concerted efforts from healthcare stakeholders, governments, and communities to ensure equitable access to excellent care and improved outcomes for those with diabetes.

Personalized Medicine Approaches

In the ever-evolving panorama of healthcare, personalized medicine emerges as a beacon of hope, ushering in a new era of focused and specialized treatment techniques. This paradigm shift is revolutionizing the way we see and address medical illnesses, and diabetes, in particular, promises to profit tremendously from this novel approach.

At its core, personalized medicine tailor's treatment strategies to each patient's unique genetic, biochemical, and behavioral traits. For individuals with diabetes, this means going beyond the standard one-size-fits-all treatment model to a more nuanced and successful approach. Genetic testing, molecular profiling, and improved diagnostic techniques enable healthcare providers to get deeper insights into a patient's genetic composition, allowing for personalized interventions that address the fundamental causes of diabetes.

One of the primary advantages of personalized medicine in diabetes care is the capacity to discover genetic markers related to disease risk and development. By understanding an individual's genetic propensity, healthcare providers can forecast susceptibility to diabetes and apply preventative interventions customized to each person's unique needs. This proactive approach not only minimizes the occurrence of diabetes but also enables individuals to make informed lifestyle choices for optimal health.

Moreover, personalized medicine extends its impact on diabetes care. Tailoring pharmaceutical regimens based on hereditary characteristics and treatment responses optimizes the efficiency of therapies, minimizing side effects and maximizing therapeutic outcomes. Precision in prescribing pharmaceutical amounts and types becomes crucial, ensuring patients receive the most suitable and effective therapies for their specific circumstances.

Beyond genetics, personalized medicine encompasses a holistic view of an individual's health profile, combining lifestyle aspects such as nutrition, physical exercise, and environmental effects. This holistic approach helps healthcare providers design individualized tactics that correspond with a patient's choices and circumstances, enabling higher adherence to treatment programs.

While personalized medicine offers a promising option for increasing diabetes care, issues such as cost, accessibility, and ethical considerations must be addressed. However, as technology continues to advance and our understanding of the intricate interplay between genetics and health deepens, personalized medicine holds the potential to revolutionize diabetes management, providing tailored solutions that prioritize individual well-being and improve overall health outcomes.

Targeting Diabetes Prevention on a Global Scale

Targeting diabetes prevention on the global level involves a multidimensional approach that tackles the numerous socioeconomic, cultural, and healthcare inequities common throughout different regions of the world. With diabetes growing as a serious public health concern affecting millions globally, concerted efforts are necessary to prevent its rising prevalence and ameliorate its impact on individuals and communities.

Education and awareness activities serve as essential pillars in global diabetes prevention efforts. Empowering individuals with knowledge about risk factors, healthy lifestyle choices, and preventive measures empowers them to make informed decisions and take proactive steps toward diabetes prevention. By boosting health knowledge and cultivating community engagement, these efforts establish the framework for sustainable preventative strategies.

Furthermore, collaboration between governments, healthcare organizations, non-profit entities, and community stakeholders is crucial to mobilize resources and implement effective preventative programs. Policies that promote healthy settings, such as access to nutritious food alternatives, safe recreational areas, and cheap healthcare services, play a key role in changing individuals' habits and preventing the onset of diabetes.

In addition to preventative interventions at the individual and community levels, addressing the socioeconomic determinants of health is crucial in worldwide diabetes prevention initiatives. Socioeconomic factors such as poverty, inequality, and lack of access to education and healthcare services strongly impact diabetes risk and outcomes. Implementing policies that address these underlying variables, such as poverty alleviation programs, social safety nets, and equitable healthcare systems, can help lower diabetes prevalence and improve health outcomes on a worldwide scale.

Harnessing technology and innovation also have enormous potential in scaling up diabetes preventive efforts internationally. Digital health solutions, mobile applications, and telemedicine platforms increase access to healthcare services, encourage health monitoring, and deliver individualized therapies, particularly in underprivileged and rural places. Moreover, combining big data analytics and artificial intelligence enables predictive modeling and targeted treatments, optimizing resource allocation and enhancing the effectiveness of prevention strategies.

Fostering relationships and knowledge-sharing among countries and international organizations is vital in promoting diabetes prevention on a global scale. Collaborative research efforts, capacity-building programs, and policy exchanges promote the exchange of best practices, lessons learned, and creative ways, accelerating progress toward the shared goal of diabetes prevention worldwide.

Targeting diabetes prevention on a global scale demands a comprehensive and collaborative approach that addresses socioeconomic gaps, improves health literacy, uses technology, and fosters international cooperation. By prioritizing preventative efforts and implementing evidence-based methods, we can lessen the growing burden of diabetes and improve health outcomes for individuals and communities worldwide.

Health Equity and Access to Diabetes Care

Achieving health equity and ensuring access to diabetes care are essential principles of healthcare systems globally. However, discrepancies in access to diabetes care exist, particularly among marginalized populations and underprivileged communities. Addressing these discrepancies needs a coordinated effort to deconstruct barriers and promote equitable access to important diabetic services.

One of the biggest hurdles to receiving diabetes care is socioeconomic disparity. Individuals from lower socioeconomic origins sometimes encounter obstacles in receiving healthcare services due to budgetary constraints, lack of health insurance coverage, and limited access to healthcare facilities. Moreover, institutional problems such as racial and ethnic prejudice, language difficulties, and geographical differences further compound these inequalities, restricting patients' capacity to get timely and quality diabetes care.

To address health equality and enhance access to diabetes care, a multi-pronged approach is needed. Firstly, legislative initiatives aiming at eliminating financial obstacles, such as expanding health insurance coverage and subsidizing diabetic drugs and supplies, can help improve the affordability and accessibility of care for underprivileged populations. Additionally, focused outreach programs and community-based initiatives can assist in bridging gaps in access by bringing healthcare services closer to underserved communities, resolving transportation hurdles, and offering culturally and linguistically appropriate care.

Furthermore, healthcare providers play a significant role in promoting health equity by implementing patient-centered approaches that prioritize the needs and preferences of diverse patient populations. Culturally competent care, which entails knowing and respecting patients' cultural beliefs, values, and practices, can promote patient-provider communication, trust, and participation, ultimately improving health outcomes among minority and underserved populations.

Innovative ways of employing technology and telemedicine can also help overcome hurdles to receiving diabetes care, particularly in remote and underserved locations. Telehealth services, mobile health software, and remote monitoring devices enable consumers to access virtual consultations, receive real-time feedback on their health condition, and remotely manage their diabetes, thereby boosting ease and accessibility of care.

Moreover, addressing social determinants of health, such as education, housing, and work, is vital in improving health equity and assuring access to diabetes care. Collaborative efforts between healthcare professionals, community organizations, and governments are needed to undertake upstream interventions that address these structural problems and build supportive settings for health.

Achieving health equity and assuring access to diabetes care needs a comprehensive and multi-sectoral approach that addresses socioeconomic inequities, structural impediments, and cultural variables affecting healthcare access. By implementing legislative initiatives, supporting culturally competent care, harnessing technology, and addressing socioeconomic determinants of health, we may promote health equality and improve diabetes outcomes for all persons, regardless of their background or circumstances.

Overcoming Barriers to Implementing Evidence-Based Strategies

Implementing evidence-based solutions in healthcare settings can be problematic due to many constraints that inhibit its adoption and incorporation into clinical practice. Identifying and overcoming these hurdles is vital to enable the effective adoption of evidence-based procedures and enhance patient outcomes.

One key hurdle to implementing evidence-based strategies is resistance to change among healthcare practitioners. Clinicians may be used to old procedures or dubious of new interventions, leading to difficulty in implementing evidence-based guidelines. Overcoming this barrier demands developing a culture of continual learning and professional growth inside healthcare institutions. Providing education and training programs, engaging clinicians in the decision-making process, and creating incentives for adopting evidence-based practices can help lessen resistance to change and build a culture of evidence-based care.

Another significant impediment is the absence of resources and infrastructure to facilitate the implementation of evidence-based methods. Healthcare institutions may confront constraints such as restricted money, poor staffing, and obsolete technology, which hinder their capacity to effectively apply evidence-based standards. Addressing these resource-related hurdles involves strategic planning and allocation of resources, including financial investments in infrastructure enhancements, personnel development, and technology adoption. Collaboration with stakeholders, including legislators, payers, and healthcare executives, is vital in lobbying for enough resources to support evidence-based practice.

Additionally, organizational culture and leadership play a key impact in promoting or obstructing the implementation of evidence-based initiatives. Strong leadership support and a healthy organizational culture that promotes innovation, teamwork, and quality improvement are crucial for effective implementation. Leaders must promote evidence-based practice, establish clear goals and expectations, and give continuing support and resources to frontline workers. Creating interdisciplinary teams and promoting collaboration among physicians, administrators, and other stakeholders can help boost the implementation process by harnessing varied perspectives and skills.

Furthermore, external considerations like as regulatory constraints, reimbursement policies, and external demands from stakeholders might influence the adoption of evidence-based practices. Healthcare companies must negotiate these external issues successfully to guarantee alignment with evidence-based guidelines while also meeting regulatory and financial needs. Advocacy activities, stakeholder involvement, and collaboration with professional organizations can assist overcome these external hurdles and create an enabling climate for evidence-based practice.

Overcoming hurdles to implementing evidence-based methods involves a multi-faceted approach that tackles organizational, cultural, resource-related, and external variables. By developing a culture of continuous learning, investing in resources and infrastructure, giving strong leadership support, and navigating external pressures effectively, healthcare organizations can successfully implement evidence-based practices and enhance patient outcomes.

In conclusion, the journey towards better diabetes treatment and management is continuous, and there are still various difficulties to overcome. However, with combined efforts from healthcare professionals, lawmakers, researchers, and community people, tremendous improvement can be made. It is crucial to acknowledge the importance of evidence-based approaches, patient-centered care, and health equity in obtaining optimal results for those living with diabetes.

Moving forward, we must continue to focus on preventative initiatives, early identification, and comprehensive approaches to diabetes management. This involves promoting healthy lifestyle practices, increasing access to screening and early intervention programs, and addressing social determinants of health that impact diabetes outcomes.

Furthermore, there is an urgent need for investment in research and innovation to discover novel treatments, technologies, and interventions that can enhance diabetes management and outcomes. This includes improving precision medical approaches, using digital health solutions, and exploring individualized treatment choices based on genetic and molecular profiles.

Moreover, lobbying for legislation and activities that support diabetes prevention, education, and access to quality care is crucial. This involves fostering health equality, addressing disparities in diabetes prevalence and outcomes, and ensuring that all individuals, regardless of socioeconomic position or geographic location, have access to the services and assistance they need to properly manage their diabetes.

In conclusion, let us continue to work collectively toward a future where diabetes care is accessible, egalitarian, and successful for all individuals. By embracing innovation, evidence-based methods, and a commitment to patient-centered care, we can make tremendous progress in improving the lives of those afflicted by diabetes and lowering the burden of this chronic disease on folks, families, and communities worldwide.

Recapitulation of Key Points

In summary, this detailed talk has highlighted numerous areas of diabetes treatment and control. We began by exploring the pathophysiology and intervention techniques for both Type 1 and Type 2 diabetes, identifying the processes underlying their development and the pharmaceutical therapies available. Lifestyle adjustments, including dietary approaches, exercise regimes, and weight management measures, were stressed as key components of diabetes care.

We dug into the relevance of psychosocial considerations and support for diabetes patients, acknowledging the impact of mental health on overall well-being. Additionally, we reviewed the numerous kinds of diabetes, including gestational diabetes, monogenic diabetes, and other unusual forms, each requiring specific approaches to control.

Furthermore, we studied the role of technology in diabetes care, including wearable devices and remote monitoring technologies, and the potential for digital health solutions to increase patient outcomes. We also discussed the issue of health equality and access to diabetes care, acknowledging the gaps that exist and the necessity for tailored initiatives to overcome them.

Additionally, we examined the obstacles associated with applying evidence-based techniques and overcoming barriers to care. Finally, we touched upon the future directions and difficulties in diabetes care, emphasizing the significance of continuous research, innovation, and advocacy efforts to improve outcomes for those living with diabetes.

Overall, this conversation underlines the varied character of diabetes care and the significance of a holistic strategy that addresses the biological, psychological, social, and environmental aspects that influence diabetes outcomes. By integrating personalized medical techniques, using technology, and prioritizing health equity, we may move towards a future where diabetes is effectively managed and its burden decreased for individuals and communities worldwide.

Importance of Evidence-Based Approaches

The importance of evidence-based healthcare practices cannot be emphasized. When it comes to managing and treating illnesses like diabetes, focusing on evidence-based methods guarantees that interventions are grounded in scientific research and proven to be beneficial. This strategy prioritizes treatments and tactics that have been carefully studied and shown to have favorable outcomes, ultimately leading to enhanced patient care and better health outcomes.

Evidence-based approaches provide healthcare practitioners with a framework for decision-making, encouraging them to select interventions that are backed by high-quality research and data. This helps to guarantee that patients receive the most appropriate and effective treatments suited to their specific needs. By adhering to evidence-based recommendations and protocols, healthcare practitioners can enhance patient care, minimize risks, and maximize the possibility of favorable results.

Furthermore, evidence-based approaches enhance accountability and openness in healthcare delivery. By basing judgments on rigorous scientific evidence, healthcare providers may justify their choices and actions, creating trust and confidence among patients and the larger community. This transparency also enables for continuing examination and refining of processes, ensuring that healthcare delivery continuously changes to accord with the latest research and best practices.

In addition to influencing clinical decision-making, evidence-based approaches play a significant role in informing healthcare policy and budget allocation. Policymakers rely on evidence-based research to influence public health efforts, provide funds, and produce guidelines that support population-wide health benefits. By picking initiatives with a good evidence base, policymakers may maximize the impact of limited resources and address the most pressing healthcare needs within communities.

Moreover, evidence-based approaches empower individuals to make educated decisions regarding their treatment. By providing patients with evidence-based information and options, healthcare practitioners enable them to actively participate in their treatment plans and take responsibility for their health. This shared decision-making approach fosters collaboration between patients and physicians, resulting in increased patient satisfaction and adherence to treatment regimens.

Evidence-based techniques are critical for delivering high-quality, effective, and patient-centered care in diabetes management and across the healthcare spectrum. By anchoring interventions in scientific research and data, healthcare professionals can maximize patient outcomes, promote transparency and accountability, inform healthcare policy, and empower individuals to take an active part in their health. As healthcare continues to evolve, supporting evidence-based approaches will remain crucial in driving positive change and improving health outcomes for individuals and communities alike.

Empowering Patients and Healthcare Providers

Empowering people and healthcare practitioners are crucial to creating collaborative and effective healthcare delivery. This approach stresses the need for active involvement from both parties in decision-making processes and treatment plans, ultimately leading to improved patient outcomes and satisfaction.

For patients, empowerment means giving them the knowledge, skills, and support they need to actively engage in their healthcare journey. This includes teaching patients about their disease, treatment alternatives, and self-management measures in a straightforward and accessible manner. By knowing their disease and treatment alternatives, patients can make educated decisions that correspond with their preferences and values, leading to improved engagement and adherence to treatment plans.

Moreover, empowering patients requires developing a collaborative partnership between patients and healthcare providers. This collaboration is built on mutual respect, trust, and open communication, where patients feel comfortable expressing their problems and desires, and healthcare providers listen attentively and provide appropriate support. By integrating patients into decision-making processes and honoring their unique needs and preferences, healthcare practitioners can boost patient satisfaction and encourage a sense of ownership over their health.

In addition to empowering patients, it is as crucial to empower healthcare providers to deliver patient-centered care successfully. This involves providing healthcare personnel with the training, resources, and support they need to engage with patients in a meaningful and empathic manner. By equipping healthcare personnel with effective communication skills, cultural competence training, and tools for collaborative decision-making, they may create trustworthy relationships with patients and deliver treatment that is responsive to patients' needs and preferences.

Further, empowering healthcare providers entails building a supportive work atmosphere that values cooperation, ongoing learning, and professional development. This includes developing a culture of teamwork and interdisciplinary collaboration, where healthcare providers work together to meet complicated patient requirements and optimize care delivery. Additionally, providing chances for continued education and training ensures that healthcare providers keep up-to-date on the latest evidence-based practices and emerging technology, enabling them to give high-quality treatment.

Empowering patients and healthcare providers is vital for obtaining optimal healthcare outcomes and increasing the patient experience. By building collaborative relationships, offering education and assistance, and creating a friendly work environment, patients and healthcare providers can work together effectively to negotiate the difficulties of healthcare delivery and enhance health outcomes. Empowering all parties ultimately leads to a more patient-centered and effective healthcare system.

Looking Ahead: Towards a Diabetes-Free Future

Looking ahead, the vision of a diabetes-free future inspires optimism and motivates innovation in the field of healthcare. While diabetes offers enormous hurdles, breakthroughs in research, technology, and public health programs offer potential paths for prevention, control, and ultimately, the eradication of this chronic disease.

As we continue to increase our understanding of the underlying mechanisms and risk factors linked with diabetes, we are better positioned to design targeted therapies and tailored treatment methods. This includes harnessing cutting-edge technology such as genetic sequencing, biomarker analysis, and artificial intelligence to identify individuals at high risk of developing diabetes and customize interventions to their specific requirements.

Furthermore, the growing emphasis on prevention through lifestyle modifications, early identification through screening programs, and access to inexpensive healthcare services holds the potential to limit the rising prevalence of diabetes internationally. By providing individuals with the knowledge and resources they need to make healthy choices and manage their health successfully, we may greatly lessen the burden of diabetes on individuals, families, and healthcare systems.

In addition to individual-level interventions, addressing the socioeconomic determinants of health and promoting health equity are key components of reaching a diabetes-free future. This involves addressing variables such as socioeconomic position, availability of healthy dietary options, safe environments for physical activity, and culturally responsive healthcare services. By addressing these underlying drivers, we may build supportive environments that enable all persons to make healthy choices and minimize their chance of getting diabetes.

Collaboration across sectors, including healthcare professionals, researchers, policymakers, community organizations, and persons affected by diabetes, is vital for driving progress toward a diabetes-free future. By working together, sharing knowledge and resources, and coordinating efforts towards common goals, we can accelerate the pace of innovation and generate sustainable change in the battle against diabetes.

In conclusion, while the route toward a diabetes-free future may be tough, it is a vision worth pursuing with determination and optimism. By utilizing breakthroughs in research, technology, and public health initiatives, and fostering collaboration across sectors, we can revolutionize the landscape of diabetes treatment and pave the path for a healthier future for generations to come. Together, we can transform the vision of a diabetes-free future into a reality.